Advance Praise for *Training for Sud*

Those of us who teach self-defense have a vital responsibility to ensure that our students can actually use what they learn. The challenge is that we can never know when a student will be forced to apply their skills. It could be today, tomorrow, next year, or never. That makes it the instructor's responsibility to make each and every student as competent as possible as quickly as possible. In *Training for Sudden Violence* Rory Miller gives exercises and training philosophy that serve this goal. Some of the drills are mental, because the author recognizes that survival is not just a physical problem. Some are simple, things you can do right now. Some, like scenarios, are on the leading edge of current professional training. There's a lot in this book, and no fluff. Concise, effective, and useful, I cannot recommend it highly enough!

—Lawrence A. Kane, martial artist, author of *Surviving Armed Assaults*, coauthor of *The Little Black Book of Violence* and *Scaling Force*

Rory Miller has once again provided a masterpiece delineating not only his well-thought-out and useful drills for martial arts and self-defense, but providing invaluable insight for teaching martial arts and self defense-skills across the broad range of experience and need. Many of his drills provide more mental and psychological training than physical and, as such, are viable to any practitioner from the novice to the expert. His book provides practical exercises building off of his previous books, *Meditations on Violence* and *Facing Violence*.

—Jeffrey Cooper, MD, emergency physician; tactical physician; sixth dan, Okinawan goju-ryu karate

Power is the ability to do things. So knowledge isn't power. Just "knowing" has no ability to get things done. Knowledge has to be effectively applied to be powerful. That's why this latest book from Rory Miller is so very important: it teaches drills that effectively develop the ability to apply many differing skills and attributes. Rory once again shares his hard-won expertise in a logical and accessible way.

—Iain Abernethy, sixth dan, World Combat Association chief international coach, author of *Mental Strength*, *Throws for Strikers*, and *Karate's Grappling Methods*

The best way to train for a serious fight is full out; however, if you do that, you may break your toys—or they may break you. If somebody doesn't get hurt, you are doing it wrong. Rory Miller has developed a series of drills that can help. No drill is perfect, but those in this book on how to survive serious mayhem are effective. Read it, and learn.

—Steve Perry, *New York Times* best-selling author, *Shadows of the Empire*

Books by Rory Miller
Meditations on Violence
Facing Violence
Force Decisions
Scaling Force
Conflict Communication

Video by Rory Miller
Facing Violence
Logic of Violence
Joint Locks
Infighting

TRAINING FOR SUDDEN VIOLENCE

TRAINING FOR SUDDEN VIOLENCE

72 Practical Drills

Rory Miller

YMAA Publication Center
Wolfeboro, NH USA

YMAA Publication Center, Inc.
Main Office:
PO Box 480
Wolfeboro, New Hampshire, 03894
1-800-669-8892 • info@ymaa.com • www.ymaa.com

ISBN: 9781594393808 (print) • ISBN: 9781594393815 (ebook)

Copyright © 2016 by Rory Miller
Edited by T. G. LaFredo
Cover design by Axie Breen
Photos courtesy of the author unless otherwise noted

20191214

Publisher's Cataloging in Publication
Names: Miller, Rory, author.
Title: Training for sudden violence : 72 practical drills / Rory Miller.
Description: Wolfeboro, NH USA : YMAA Publication Center, [2016] | Includes biblio-
    graphical references and index.
Identifiers: ISBN: 978-1-59439-380-8 | 978-1-59439-381-5 (ebook) | LCCN: 2016941588
Subjects: LCSH: Self-defense—Handbooks, manuals, etc. | Self-defense—Psychological
    aspects. | Violence—Psychological aspects. | Violence—Prevention—Handbooks, man-
    uals, etc. | Crime prevention—Handbooks, manuals, etc. | Martial arts—Handbooks,
    manuals, etc. | Martial arts—Psychological aspects. | Fighting (Psychology) | Criminal
    psychology. | BISAC: SPORTS & RECREATION / Martial Arts & Self-Defense. |
    SOCIAL SCIENCE / Criminology. | SOCIAL SCIENCE / Violence in Society.
Classification: LCC: GV1111.M5572016 | DDC: 613.6/6—   dc23

Dedicated to the Memory of Tim Bown
1977–2010
An extraordinary friend, teacher, father, and husband.
Also the best scenario role-player
it has ever been my privilege to work with.
Rest well, brother.

CONTENTS

FOREWORD

Wim Demeere

Before I talk about this book, I need to mention a couple of things.

First of all: mankind is violent. It always has been, and it probably always will be. As a species, one of the few constants in our history is the presence of violence. Be it one on one or between tribes, cities, countries, or coalitions of nations, we've been fighting among ourselves for thousands of years.

At a personal level, there are varying reasons or pretexts as to why they come to blows:

- Bashing somebody's head in to steal his money, clothes, or other valuables.

- Defending a real or perceived insult to your honor or the honor of your wife, family, or clan.

- Your emotions get the better of you in a heated argument, and you let a punch fly.

- There are many more, but for the most part, these reasons have not changed all that much throughout time. What *has* changed is society.

In the average Western country, violence is actually much less prevalent than it was a mere hundred or two hundred years ago in that exact same place. To put this in the proper context, ask yourself these questions:

- When was the last time bandits raided your town to loot, plunder, and rape?

- When was the last time you had to shoot or kill somebody to defend your family from being murdered by robbers?

- When was the last time you lost a family member to a lynch mob?

Once again, the list is much longer, but for most Westerners, the answer to these questions is "Never." Just the questions themselves seem absurd to them, even though these things were a part of daily life not that long ago. This doesn't mean violence is nonexistent in today's societies—on the contrary. It is still a part of life, but in many cases you can avoid it; in only a very few instances will an aggressor follow you all the way home if you successfully run away from him.

As a consequence, very few people have any actual experience with or accurate knowledge of dealing with violence. For the most part, they get their information on this topic from television shows and movies. Unfortunately, those are perhaps the worst possible sources you can turn to for realistic information on this subject. As a result, people no longer have the skills to cope with violence, regardless of what form it takes.

This informational void has given the opportunity to countless experts to offer their advice on this problem via books, videos, and training programs. Sometimes they offer worthwhile information; more often, the opposite is the case. But the average civilian no longer has the means to separate the good from the bad, as he lacks a realistic empirical framework to do so. This, in turn, has allowed a large number of unrealistic and inefficient teachings to flourish. Along with that, there is the omnipresence of the internet, which allows every single person with a computer to spread the most outlandish ideas on violence.

Just as the glossy magazines have indoctrinated women worldwide to strive for a size four regardless of their body type, this avalanche of faulty information on violence has become part of the collective unconscious.

One of those erroneous ideas is that training drills are useless for self-defense. Though there are indeed some popular drills that offer little of value, nothing could be further from the truth. Warriors, soldiers, and all those who routinely engage in violence have always used drills to hone their skills:

Roman soldiers started their sword training by relentlessly drilling techniques on a wooden post. They were not allowed to practice swordplay with a partner until they had mastered those drills.

"Tent pegging" (piercing and picking up a ground target with a sword or spear while riding in gallop) was practiced by cavalries in Asia and Europe since at least 400 BC.

- The sport of polo originated from another ancient drill for cavalries to practice sword techniques while on horseback.
- Friedrich von Steuben insisted on bayonet training drills during the American Revolutionary War, and they proved decisive on the battlefield.

If warriors from those times, when life was significantly more violent than today, understood the value of training drills, then we should probably do the same today. The only question that remains is, which drills should we use?

That is where this book comes in.

Having trained, sparred, and talked with Rory, I can state from firsthand experience that he definitely knows what he writes about. He has a unique blend of formal and informal training in both martial arts and law enforcement, vast experience in handling extremely violent conflicts, and a sharp analytical mind. All these factors combined make his knowledge and insight invaluable when creating drills or adapting existing ones so they become more effective. With this book, he has done exactly that.

Some of the drills are tried and tested; they've stood the test of time, and many instructors use them because they work so well. Others are variations of these drills where Rory made some changes that increased the benefits you derive from them. Many others will be brand new to you, as they are not commonly used in most schools or dojos. But the most valuable thing you will get out of this book is the drill that blows you away and that creates a lasting paradigm shift for not only your training but also for how you view violence. I'm confident you will find at the very least several such drills here.

What is perhaps just as important is how Rory explains the drills in such a way that you can tweak them for your own purposes and specific circumstances. This is the hallmark of powerful training tools: they are versatile enough to be adapted to each individual's needs. This also means you can continue to get more and more out of the drills in this book as your own skills increase because of your training.

Violence is a huge and complex topic. Training to handle violence is the same, perhaps even more so. The information in this book is a practical guide to help you on that path. I hope you can get just as much out of it as I did.

Enjoy your training,
Wim Demeere
Former Belgian *sanda* champion, personal trainer, author . . . and about 220 pounds of solid muscle and skill we lovingly refer to as the BBBB (the Big Blond Belgian Bastard)

INTRODUCTION

I teach about violence. I worked in corrections for the better part of two decades, and as I left "the life" I discovered that my niche wasn't so much teaching cops, as I had expected, or even teaching civilian self-defense. The material seemed to resonate most with experienced martial artists who were coming to discover how little they really knew about violence.

The first book, *Meditations on Violence* (YMAA, 2008), was as much therapy and catharsis as information. It was a mental dump of what I knew about Bad Stuff™.

The second, *Facing Violence* (YMAA, 2011), is less visceral and far less personal. But it is, in my opinion, far more useful. How to read a room, how to identify and classify violent people and situations, the nuances of explaining a split-second decision in logical, legal terms.

This one will be different. Maija Soderholm, author of *The Liar, the Cheat, and the Thief* and one of the sneakiest swordswomen I know, suggested a book of drills and exercises. Things that are suited to my goal (surviving violence) and to my way of teaching, which is getting the student to see and evaluate clearly enough that each student becomes a self-teacher.

Teaching, especially in martial arts, is often hierarchical. There is a clear sense of who is above and who is below. Information flows down, always under control of the instructor. Sometimes it comes with a ritual of dominance and submission: some students bow to a master.

I believe that you cannot be taught simultaneously to bow and to stand your ground. That the habit of obedience is a short step away from the habit of submission. That if you do what your instructor says when you know in your heart it is wrong, you will also obey a rapist. Trust me, a violent predator is far scarier than your instructor. Maybe not on an intellectual level ("My instructor kicks ass! He is the best fighter I have ever seen"). But on a gut level ("This man is going to hurt me and hurt me and he is never going to stop and he is enjoying every second").

It's not that criminals are somehow magically better fighters than people who train and stay in shape. It is that criminals will go to a place inside themselves that your instructor will not, a place that too many people cannot even imagine.

So what follows are drills and exercises that I think are important for observation, for integrating mind/body, and for efficient motion.

Some involve motion, because anything that escalates to a physical fight is a matter of motion. Many involve mind-set, because most of the catastrophic failures I have seen in a fight have been mental, not physical. Almost all, at some level, are about accurately seeing the world.

I believe there are three aspects you must master to successfully defend yourself: awareness, initiative, and permission.

Awareness is as broad and deep or as narrow and focused as you can handle it. From seeing in an instant the position and momentum of an attacker and each part of the attacker to seeing the dynamics of a room or a street, awareness goes as far as you have the discipline and curiosity to take it. It must be an informed awareness, however. Seeing everything is not the same as understanding everything. You may notice three young men suddenly going silent and separating, but if you do not recognize what that means, the information is useless.

Initiative is the ability to act decisively and ruthlessly. Simply to act. Simply to move. Make a decision. Execute.

People hesitate. They make a decision and they question it. They decide to move and then they prepare to move and set to move. All of these hesitations are visible and take time. They make you an easier victim.

Permission is the ability to do what you have decided to do. You have an entire lifetime of social conditioning telling you what conflict is and how to deal with it. When the type of violence you are facing is different from the social conflict you have been prepared for, the social responses *will not work*. Not only do violent criminals know this, they count on it. You must give yourself permission to break the rules, and to do that, you must know what the rules are.

There are also four elements in any conflict: you, the threat or threats (bad guys), the environment, and luck.

Most martial arts are centered on *you*: teaching you to move, to punch, kick, pin, and throw. Further, much of the training focuses on the physical self and at best pays lip service to the ethical, spiritual, emotional, and intellectual aspects. You have a brain and a spirit that must be explored and trained. All three (mind, body, spirit) are potential points of failure. You must emphasize the strengths and know the weaknesses.

There is also a *bad guy* (or many) in a fight, and you must understand him. If he is a predator, he is there neither to test you nor to help you develop skills. He is there to take something from you and do it as safely and efficiently as possible. To let you know anything in advance or to feed you the type of attacks you have trained against would be stupid. Do not count on the threat being stupid. You should know, as much as possible, how threats think and feel and plan as well as how all humans move and how they break.

Fights happen in *places*. Often, training is set up to minimize the variables of environment so specific skills can be trained and tested. It is fine as long as you understand the depth of the limitation. You will fight in a world of infinite hazards and opportunities. The one who is better at seeing and exploiting these has a huge edge in the real world.

Last is *luck*. Professionals work to take luck out of any planned operations and dojo are kept clean and uncluttered to try to minimize chaos. Chaos is the natural environment of a fight. Stuff happens. What you don't see, like slippery surfaces or a table behind you, can have a profound effect on the outcome. Managing chaos, the use and mitigation of luck, is a skill as well—a skill centered on awareness of possibility or hazard and ruthless exploitation (e.g., initiative) of those elements.

Fighting is inherently conservative and this shows in martial arts. Fighting is dangerous. People get hurt and killed. For everything that might work, there are a hundred things that seem like a good idea that can lead to a messy death. We have kata and tradition *not* because people are stuck in tradition, but because when people consistently survived, it was considered imperative to remember how and model it.

A lot has been lost in translation and by transmission over time, but most of the systems that survived have the bones. But that may not be enough. They also were built around specific individuals in specific times and places.

> There isn't a section on training kata in this book, largely because I am not convinced kata is good training for assault survival. I think kata was the premier way to preserve and transmit physical information in a society where literacy was rare and video unheard of.

How you will fight must be built around *you*. Your physicality (both in build and in how you naturally move) as well as your temperament. A certain amount of aggression is required, but if you really cannot injure another person, training to injure is wasted time. If you can't handle messy liquid spills, knife training probably isn't for you.

I don't like the term "fighting," but I wind up using it a lot. Our obsession with social conflict and the fact that most of our experience centers in social conflict have stunted our language. So I use "fight" as a generic term, and that is very, very wrong. It puts images in your head that do not belong there.

Most conflict is social and establishes membership, establishes dominance, or enforces rules. There is no difference between a fraternity hazing and a gang "jumping in." All over the world, young men follow the same steps leading up to a fistfight. The dynamics behind a spanking and an execution are the same.

It all has rules; it all has rituals. There is a lead-up. One or both of the people usually must be angry or make themselves angry—very few people can fight "cold."

This is what we are used to. This is the default belief about violence. This is the place where "fighting," with its implications of a contest with a winner and a loser, is valid.

These assumptions drive most of our training. From the lethal duels of bygone eras to sparring today, this is what we expect and this is what we train for.

And almost every last incident of this kind of physical fight is 100 percent preventable. You can walk away from it all. All of your training works here and none of it is necessary.

Assaults are rare, but they are the most serious person-to-person attacks. A human predator wants something from you: your money and jewelry or just a few minutes of pleasure hurting you. He will get it with minimal risk to himself. Minimum effort expended.

We do not work ourselves up or get angry to slaughter a steer. An experienced criminal will not do so with you. We do not take risks or even consider somehow "making it fair" when we butcher a chicken. A predator will not play fair with you.

To make it safe and efficient for himself, the predator will make the attack close range, hard, fast, and a surprise for you.

It will be nothing like sparring. Nothing like even the most extreme no-holds-barred match.

This will be an assault, and the things you need to train for, the things I teach, are those little skills that buy you some precious warning or a microsecond. The things that might give you a few percentage points of an edge.

If you already train martial arts, nothing here (nothing in anything I teach) is intended to replace your training. Hopefully, you will find drills in here that put your training into real-world context. Exercises that will bring your mind to the pitch that hard training has brought your body. Things that will make skills a little easier to access under stress and ways to practice making the motions you have trained natural for you.

This is a book of drills and exercises. As such, it depends on certain shared concepts. You won't get the underlying concepts here. If you don't understand self-defense law or you have no idea of how bad guys attack, or the psychological and legal implications that follow a violent event are mysteries . . . well, you and I probably aren't talking about the same thing when we say "self-defense."

I also think it's kind of rude to spend a bunch of pages in a book just recapping a previous book. So here's the deal. Most of the stuff in here will be useful no matter how you study (and believe me, *how* you train is far more relevant than *what* you train). If you don't understand the relevance of something, you might want to take a look at a previous book. If the thing you don't get appears to be emotional or internal, probably *Meditations on Violence*. If the glitch is more concrete (self-defense law or different classifications of bad guys, for instance), there is probably more material in *Facing Violence*.

I suppose, for most people, martial arts and self-defense, training for violence, is something of a hobby. They do it for fun, a couple of times a week and, to my eyes, with no sense of urgency. For the last couple of years, I've been teaching mostly civilians, for the decade before that, I was teaching corrections and enforcement officers.

Every class I taught I would look at the officers and know, without a doubt, at least a third of that class would need what I taught before the year was out, and at least one would bet his or her life on it. If I bullshitted them, if I lied to them, if I made them comfortable instead of effective, the price would be paid in blood and I would be one of the ones going to do the hospital visits or, gods forfend, the funerals.

It's a huge responsibility. I had these men and women for as little as eight hours a year. Not all were in great shape: some old, some small, many had old injuries. They had to be able to prevail against younger, stronger people, people who sometimes got the first move at close range and had no compunction about spilling blood.

That responsibility forces you to rethink everything you do. You don't have time for egos. The drills aren't about identity. You know what I mean: the constant internet bickering about which style is right or whether boxing punches or karate punches are "proper."

Going home to your family is your identity. There is no time to waste. And you can't hand wave past the bad stuff. With only those eight hours we had people handle situations that experienced martial artists put in a "That's a no-win situation. We don't train for that" category.

We didn't have that option. If we took that attitude . . . hospital visits. Funerals. I hate funerals.

The pressure to make something effective, the responsibility for other people's lives, the limited time, the high stakes forced us to apply the same idea of ruthless efficiency to teaching that your martial arts should apply to combat. And it worked.

So here's my philosophy for teaching self-defense:

1. I have no interest in teaching you to do what I do. You aren't me. We have different bodies and different minds. Imitate an instructor and the best you can ever hope for is to become a flawed clone of someone else.

   But work on *you*, and you can become better than your teacher. Not the same, better. The key is to become the most efficient "you" that you can be. If you ever need these skills, I won't be there. Neither will your sensei or your mommy. Whatever saves your life must come from inside . . . so start working on your insides.

2. The physical skills of self-defense are easy. It is not that hard to kill or cripple a human being. Knowing when such force is appropriate and necessary, recognizing danger, and summoning the will to cross that line—those are rarely taught and absolutely critical.

3. The baseline of self-defense has almost no relationship to the baseline for martial arts, however. Two examples:

Let's start with one very simple thing—power generation.

A traditional martial artist is taught how to hit hard. Different systems have different methods of power generation, but two of the most common involve a solid connection with the ground and good structure.

The solid connection with the ground allows you to put the power of your legs into a punch. Good structure keeps that power from being lost or bled off into space by excessive motion. You can add more to it, whipping action with the hips and rotational power transmitted through the spine . . . doesn't matter. If you've been training for any length of time, you should have been taught how to hit hard.

Here's where it gets ugly. You get surprised.

"Not me! I have good situational awareness!" Get over that. Assuming (1) there is an experienced bad guy in the picture, and (2) you aren't creating a situation yourself—you will be surprised. If the bad guy can't get surprise, he'll go hit someone else.

Got that? If you aren't surprised, you don't get to use your skills.

You are surprised. It's not like the timing in sparring, with the closing distance and maintaining defense and some feints for you to read and interpret. Nope. The bad guy got close, got you distracted for a second, and hit

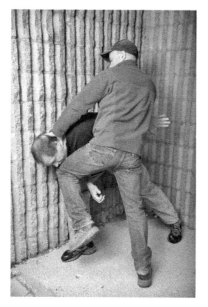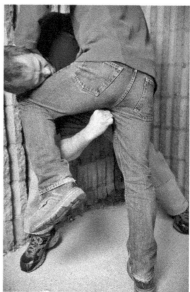

Power generation. How do you hit hard bent over, pushed into a wall, on a threat who is too close? When your connection with the ground is iffy, your structure is completely destroyed, and the blows coming at your head are making you flinch?

you. Not the one-half-power-hit-and-judge-for-effect that most inexperienced people do. Nope, it's a flurry attack, so many things coming at your face and body so fast that your mind freezes. Crunching noises and pain coming from your face, your belly collapses with a blow, and you can't breathe and you're shoved, bent over into a wall with more hits coming in.

This is the natural environment of a sudden assault, and if you don't have an answer for this situation, you don't have an answer at all.

That's just one example, but everything else in self-defense—the timing, distance, speed, strategy, targeting—is vastly different from the assumptions of sparring.

In case you don't get it yet, one more example:

At the 2011 Montreal seminar I asked, "Who is your nightmare opponent?" Take a few minutes and think about that.

One of the answers: "He'd be about 50 percent more than I weigh, much stronger, with more skill and experience."

Yeah, that would suck, huh? Then add that he gets the first move at the time and place of his choosing. And he may be counting on a previous relationship with you to keep you from acting.

Guys, our worst nightmare is where the average woman starts her day. As guys, we've been roughhousing, pushing, and hitting one another since childhood and, largely, we've been encouraged. Sometimes overtly, but often subtly, girls have been punished when they wanted to play like that. So the average man reaches adulthood (even with no formal training) better trained and far more conditioned and experienced with violence than almost any woman.

And men are stronger. We rarely get into contests of direct strength with women without holding back a lot, but when we do, the difference is stark. On top of it all, most women have only learned social strategies to deal with conflict . . . and social strategies not only fail but backfire when attempted on a predator.

Women are an easy example, but this is the baseline of self-defense. If the predator can't stack advantages to this level, he just picks someone else.

What you can do within your own weight class is irrelevant to self-defense skills. This is the baseline. This is what I train for.

EVALUATING DRILLS

I'm not a big fan of most drills. There is a fine line, but conditioned reflexes are crucial in a fight, and habits will get you killed.

Conditioned reflexes are things you do without thinking. They are essentially trained flinch responses. If something suddenly comes at your eyes you *will* do something: block, move your head, or, at the very minimum, blink. The more you train, the more sophisticated the conditioned reflex can become.

Habits are also things you do without thinking. Ways of moving. Ways of approaching problems, and even ways of thinking and seeing. Habits can be ways of thinking *without* thinking. If you always problem-solve by breaking things down into bite-sized pieces, something that began as a strategy becomes a habit, and the second it becomes a habit, you forget to look at other ways.

Habits are especially pernicious in self-defense training. In the end, a martial artist is training to break another human being. The essence of martial arts is the manufacture of corpses and cripples. In every drill designed to break a bone, if no bone breaks, there is something wrong with the drill. Something deliberately flawed to make the drill safe. You must recognize the flaw. Because with every repetition you are instilling the flaw along with the technique.

Do you pull your punches? Then missing has become a habit. Do you use three-move defenses against single-move attacks? If so, congratulations. You are well trained to beat someone who is only a third of your speed.

When you analyze any force-on-force drill (any drill where you are simulating attacking or being attacked), you first have to examine why no one is being crippled or killed. Not merely hurt, because people are lazy and cunning and will decide that pain is "close enough" and use it as an excuse to look no deeper. *Crippled or killed.*

Most likely it will be one of four things (these, of course, are the four elements that need to be done properly to cripple or kill):

1. Powder-puffing. Power generation is absent. Sometimes the power is deliberately pulled, and you make only light contact. But there is another way, too, where the "chain of power" is deliberately broken.

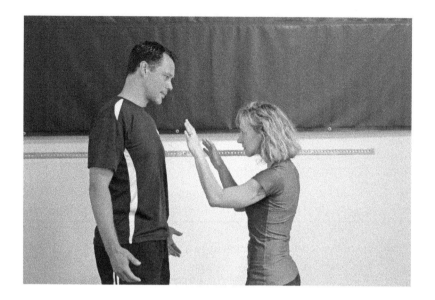

Power comes, in the end, from your feet. If you were floating weightless and struck someone, only half the power would transmit to his body. The other half would push you away as well . . . and any power that went to moving his body would also be lost, not contributing to damage.

The power chain in a hand strike comes from the feet, then up the leg bones to the pelvis, spine, and shoulder, and out the arm bones to the hands. That probably sounds esoteric. Hit a heavy bag as hard as you can. Pay attention to where your feet, hips, spine, shoulder, and arms are at the instant of impact.

If you are not using a similar alignment in the force-on-force drills, you are hitting weakly, you are hitting weakly on purpose, and you are training yourself to hit weakly under stress.

2. Targeting. If you do not use valid targets in training, you are practicing missing. Whether it is pulling strikes or using a worthless target near a good one (such as simulating eye pokes on the forehead or groin strikes on the thigh), it doesn't matter. Missing becomes a habit.

3. Ranging. This third possibility disrupts both targeting and the fourth element, timing. You cannot hit something you cannot reach. When you practice from a distance that a bad guy will not choose

(remember he wants to hurt you decisively early, so he will be close), you not only hamper your ability to do harm but throw off your own senses of safety, distance, and timing.

Defensively, working out of range gives you more time than you will have in a real assault. Because you are safe, it lacks the intensity of the real thing. Years of practicing against feeds leave the practitioner totally unprepared for attacks.

A feed may have a similar motion to a punch or stab, but it is designed and delivered specifically to be defeated. A little slow, on a known line, maybe slightly overextended or held out for just a second. No matter how much it looks like a punch, almost every element is different in a fight . . . and so people who have practiced against feeds are often completely blown away by the intensity, speed, ferocity, and pain of a "simple" attack.

4. Timing. This is the flaw I incorporate most often, because I have never seen anyone go slow motion in a real fight. Not move at all, completely frozen? Yes. I've seen that, but not slow motion.

It is still a serious flaw because it may set the expectation that there will be time to think.

Safety is not the only cause of flaws that creep into the drill. People want to win, they want to be dominant, especially if they are teaching from ego, and they want the techniques to work.

So in slow-motion drills, one speeds up so that he can win. Or the technique is taught against a slow thrust from too far away, giving the defender enough time to do the technique.

When Bo and I were going for our *mokuroku* certificates, our kata had gone through a progression until we were practicing full force and speed with bokken. We were told explicitly that to do it any other way would give *tori*, the defender, bad timing and bad skills. It was dangerous but very good training.

I was asked to be *uke*, the attacker, for a mokuroku test at another school. Same system, different instructor. First practice night I attacked the way I had been taught . . . and clocked the mokuroku candidate upside the head. The head sensei took me aside and chewed me out. He said, "At your rank, you should know that it is uke's responsibility to make tori look good. You need to slow down and be sure to fall big. I don't care if he misses completely. Making him look good is tori's job."

At my rank in my school, uke's job was to give the most realistic attack possible.

Most damning is when the student must be taught, even brainwashed, for the techniques to work. We've all seen students throwing themselves. We've seen, in real life or in parody, instructors who insist on one type of attack, the type of attack that their defenses work against. Here are the clues to look for:

1. If the uke (I'll use that term for "demonstration dummy" in this context) must be told what will happen, being told is likely part of the technique. People are largely suggestible, and if someone with sufficient authority tells you that slap at point X will cause the arm to go numb or a temporary loss of consciousness, many people will experience it. Strangely enough, it often doesn't work without the explanation, and that's something you can test.

2. If you see the technique fail on strangers, if the demonstrator must use his own students in order to demonstrate, it likely won't work on attackers either.

Most techniques in martial arts are not practiced against attacks. They are practiced against feeds.

So, to recap:

When examining a drill, first look for the safety flaw.

Then ask yourself: If the attack came at full speed and intensity, would my response work? Does it require me to have super speed or to block a full-power thrust with a thumb?

Then the third question: If I were a criminal and not stupid, would I ever do an attack this way?

That's important. Unless you plan on getting into duels, you will be attacked by a criminal, not a competitor. This is what the criminal does as a job. And he does it to maximize his safety, which means he will minimize your chances.

Enraged people do attack stupidly, and there is value in working defenses to rage attacks. Definitely practice for that . . . but if you look at an attack and just can't see a bad guy doing it, you're probably wasting your time.

The fourth question: Is this going to get me killed?

Not too long ago I was practicing *hubud*, a Filipino drill, with an advanced practitioner. Knife comes in, check, slash the arm, transition maintaining the check, slash at him . . .

He got irate. "You have to let my weapon hand go when it is my turn. That is how the drill works!"

"But that would be stupid."

I get especially annoyed with weapons. Unarmed defense against a weapon sucks, and there is no room for filling one's head with bullshit. Never, ever, ever practice dying and do not train to be killed. The stakes are too high to blindly imprint a habit, even a habit as simple as handing a weapon back once you have disarmed someone.

If the drill requires you to miss or to give up control of a weapon—or to give up a good position to transition to one that may or may not be better—or any other stupid thing that could get you killed . . . it is a bad drill.

Let me be clear. There is no way to exactly replicate breaking people without breaking them. In unarmed arts, with no weapon to "make safe," the techniques themselves have been altered. Unless the students and teachers are very aware, this alteration becomes the "right" way to do the technique.

Look for these:

1) When the drill sets an unrealistic expectation of what an attack will be like, such as practicing against long-range, slow knife thrusts when we know that shankings happen close, quickly, and from the side.

2) When the drill allows techniques that would be unsafe or crippling for the person using them in real life. It used to be a common story in fencing that the lunge was a modern invention. It wasn't that the old duelists hadn't thought of lunging; it turns out that on wet grass, the lunge is a damn good way to tear out your groin muscles.

The MMA competitor who tries a shoot on concrete and breaks his patella.

3) Most damning, when the solution to the drill is based on the *flaw*, such as using medium-speed defenses to defeat slow-motion attacks.

Coming from a Western background for weapons arts (fencing, primarily), I was taught that Western students come to training with *the* three worst habits in weapon fighting: they stay out of range, they aim at the opposing weapon instead of the opponent, and their rhythms are predictable. I was taught that these were the absolute worst habits with a weapon. And we always blamed the choreographed sword fights on television for these flaws.

So I refuse to do *sinawali* (a Filipino figure-eight-pattern partner drill). Every last aspect of it is a bad habit.

It is practiced from out of range. If I can only hit his weapon, not him, I don't swing. Striking a weapon is rarely a good idea unless you are sure you have a superior weapon . . . and if someone wants to swing while you are out of range, let him.

It works in long sweeps, high/low, when the impact in the middle could be ridden to give a harder, faster strike to a better target.

It is predictable and there are few surer ways to be destroyed than to be the most predictable one in a fight.

Even the vaunted rhythm training: So what? Rhythm is no advantage whatsoever in an assault. Assaults are brutal, staccato—the only place for flow is in the loser's blood.

But the drill is safe. And entertaining. And makes some students feel like they are gaining a valuable skill. They are certainly ingraining something.

Instructors must know the difference between training and conditioning. I don't use conditioning here to mean strength and endurance training. Conditioning in the sense that behavioral psychology uses the term.

Both are types of teaching, getting information into a brain with the goal of affecting and improving performance. Training is where most instructors spend most of their conscious time. When you are teaching students what to do for punches, or how to kick or how to scissor legs to roll to a mount, you are training.

Conditioning happens at a deeper level of the brain. It is rarely conscious for the instructor or the student. The hindbrain sees what works and what doesn't and reinforces the habits that work. What you train may or may not come out in a fight. What you condition will, good or bad.

If you practice high-speed multiple-opponent scenarios, you are training some very good stuff: continuous movement, the geometry of multiple opponents, how to use people as environmental weapons, exploiting momentum, elements of timing, and tactical thinking.

But (unless you are using armor, and even then . . .) for safety, you are probably limiting contact. You are *learning* good things. You are *conditioning* not hitting. Conditioning goes deeper than learning.

Many good Japanese jujutsu schools practice free randori that is essentially no-holds-barred, but limited contact. They *learn* to integrate offense and defense, to use strikes, locks, gouges, takedowns, and grappling as extensions of each other. . . .

But the hindbrain notices that strikes (controlled contact) never end a match. Only submissions. *Conditioning* the students to favor grappling.

Last example: In noncontact schools, if someone makes face contact, everything stops and the student apologizes. The conditioning is that hitting people in the face is wrong. If hitting people in the head is a core of the system, conditioning comes into direct conflict with training. Almost always, under stress, conditioning, not training, rises to the surface.

Contrast that with a school that trains even a focus mitt drill where the partner tags the student and the student unleashes a flurry of aggressive, forward-pressure strikes. That conditioning is in line with training.

As an instructor, it is your responsibility to evaluate your drills and keep an eye out for any accidental conditioning.

THE ONE-STEP

The one-step arose as a useful accident. Many years ago I was reading George Mattson's *The Way of Karate* and I completely misunderstood his description of *ippon kumite*. I thought, "That's brilliant—unscripted but safe, just looking at this whole thing as a meat geometry problem . . ."

I had completely missed that ippon kumite is in fact a scripted drill. I'm not that bright. But it was a very useful failure. After all, if you're going to fall, try to fall up.

The One-Step OS

The quest for the most efficient action.

This is my most basic drill. I find it useful and versatile on many levels. At its most basic, it is very simple: one partner initiates a move in slow motion and the other partner at equal speed makes one motion to respond. The partners continue this without resetting, winding up wherever they wind up and finding solutions.

Naturally, the details get more complicated.

The flaw in this drill is the artificiality of timing—both slow motion and taking turns. Because of that, the students can and should go all out with body mechanics and targeting—perfect alignment and structure so each strike pushes through the opponent and targeted to the best options. The drill should be done so slowly that the participants can press directly on eyes or throats.

Safety concerns:

- The partners must communicate. They must all understand and respond to tapping out, as well as safe words and even utterances. "Ouch! Knock it off, you jerk!" Means exactly the same thing as a tap.

- The partners must not get competitive. If they do, injuries are likely to result. The deeper reason is that survival fighting is not competitive. In a self-defense situation, you need to get out safely. Sometimes that means neutralizing the threat. It never means dominating the threat or teaching him a lesson or showing who is the better man. Those are social games. The bad guy needs to fail. There is no advantage in his knowing that you beat him.

- There will be a tendency to speed up. Because of the precise targeting, this either becomes unsafe or, if it stays safe, reinforces bad habits, like practicing missing.

- No live weapons in the training area at any time. No guns, even unloaded ones and no sharpened knives. Blueguns and blade trainers are acceptable. The nature of the game encourages people to find opportunities in the environment. I expect my students to draw and use any weapon they notice on *you*. That would be very bad if it were a loaded gun or a real knife.

- If working with a mixed group where some are not trained to fall, instruct students to notice when balance is broken and things will go to the ground. Then the person who would fall lies down in the position he would naturally land in and the opponent assumes the position she would have at the end of the takedown. Then they continue from there.

One-step can be conducted safely with people from extremely different systems. It is a great way to learn a little bit about how someone new thinks and acts. It requires no training whatsoever—complete novices can often hang with experienced martial artists. Most importantly, it is not dependent on style and there is no rote learning to it.

It allows you to train a student with respect to the student's natural movement and mentality.

It also becomes a tool where the students can begin to think and teach themselves.

The simplicity is that as you initiate a move, your partner is looking for the most efficient thing he can possibly do. As he chooses and acts, you must come up with the most efficient thing you can possibly do with respect to his current position and motion. The "taking turns" is not about letting the other person move but about practicing on a moving, unpredictable target.

Limiting yourself to one motion forces you to find something more efficient.

Note well: each person gets one action. Not one block and one strike. One action. Block-and-strike, even simultaneous block-and-strike are sparring or dueling artifacts. Assaults happen in a flurry of damage. In order to make a simultaneous block and strike work, you would have to be not only twice as fast as the threat but also have reactions that were faster than actions. The math doesn't work. It is something we get away with because we have been practicing against feeds, not attacks. This drill will help break that habit.

Subnote: covering and striking or moving and striking are not two moves. If you have trained footwork with your strikes or trained to, say, cover your groin when going for a high kick, those are simply part of the move. The difference in blocking and striking is that both the block and the strike must be aimed and then executed. They are two separate actions because they are two separate thoughts.

Coaching tips:

- To reinforce that this drill is about self-teaching, I break every few minutes when we first start and have the students tell me what they've noticed and what they've learned. One of the first ones that come up is "You can't win on defense." If you block an incoming strike, your opponent is free to make another attack.

- If someone gets in an untenable position, have the partners maintain position, have them ease up any pressure causing pain, and have them think of options. Bad guys don't give do-overs; don't practice them here.

- Do not practice dying either. Students will have a tendency to reset and start over when they feel a decisive blow has landed. This is a bad habit. You may be knocked out in real life, but you might not. If a man can take ten bullets to the chest and head and keep fighting, it seems a little delusional (and a terrible habit) to give up over a slow-motion strike.

- It's hard to stick to one-step on the ground because so many grapplers practice a flow of motion. Try to restrict them anyway. Limiting it to one move, you often find an efficient strike that is missed when people go into grappling mode.

- Most locks are relatively complicated and take several moves to get, and thus usually fail on moving people in real life. Show how locks in real life are based on "gifts" where the threat puts himself in the lock position. By just applying power to one point, efficiently, you can make a lock work. Same goes for many takedowns.

- If two students are starting to spar, have them start with the initial attack coming from behind or on the flank.

- When a student gets stuck, have him freeze and brainstorm; then ask his partner for ideas, then other students, then the instructor.

I have seen few if any positions so hopeless that a room full of people couldn't come up with options.

o   Watch for people who are moving arms but not feet.

o   Show that striking and off-balancing are both good options.

o   It's OK to run away.

o   After they have practiced for a while, explain that they are on a quest for the golden move. The golden move is anything that prevents damage to you, causes damage to the threat, puts you in a better position, and puts the threat in a worse position all with a single motion. If every action does all four things, you will do very well.

> The golden move: a single motion that protects you from damage, damages the threat, improves your position, and worsens the threat's position.
> Simply running away can do three out of four, and that isn't bad.

• In a seminar situation, encourage students to play with people they do not know and to switch partners each time.

• Use foam "bricks" and scatter them around the training area. When a group or pair goes to the ground, they can use the brick as an equalizer. It tends to change the ground game quite a bit.

• Stop-action critique: Straight-up coaching for the one-step is dead simple: "Freeze. Go back one move. Why didn't you . . . ?" when you see an opportunity for something more efficient than whatever the student used. Don't overdo it, though, or you'll be stopping them with every move. Let them play.

• Let the rounds go for a minute or longer. At the end ask, "What did you notice? What did you learn?" And get the students to evaluate their own learning process and milk the experience for themselves. This is critical!

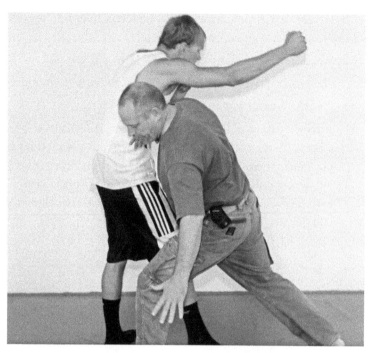

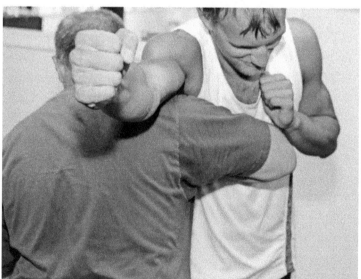

Trailing elbow drop step to a punch

It is crucial to impress on the students that the one-step is not fighting. Like most drills, it lacks the fear and pain that make fighting what fighting is. There is no test of heart in the drill and fighting is very much about determination and all those other things we call "heart."

Its purpose is to continuously move more efficiently. To find the smallest, fastest option that will get you what you want. A right hook may get the threat down (and may get your hand broken), but sometimes a two-inch popping movement with your knee can put him down as well, faster, more reliably, and more safely. But you can only do it if you see the opportunity.

In the end, this drill is about learning to see.

Four-Option One-Step

One of the paradigms I teach is movement/pain/damage/shock, or MPDS. Your combative options in any given situation can have only a few classes of effects: You can move the threat or part of the threat (clearing an arm away for an opening, pushing, rolling, or immobilizing). You can cause pain, through joint locks, pressure points, or distracting strikes. You can cause damage by striking to break bones, concussing the brain, taking a joint lock to a break, damaging organs, or disrupting the sensory system. Or you can shut down the complete system by strangulation, crushing the airway, causing internal bleeding, disrupting respiration, causing severe concussion, or compromising the cervical spine.

These four elements correspond roughly to the use-of-force continuum as trained by many force professionals:

If you can get away or make the other get away, you don't have to hurt the threat. If pain alone can make the threat stop, you don't escalate to damage. If damage can be done quickly and safely enough to make the threat stop, you don't use deadly force.

"Deadly force" is a legal concept and you want to look at your state statutes before defining it to your students.

Since the MPDS paradigm dovetails well with some of the legal concepts of self-defense, it makes a nice drill to help students understand those concepts and exercise judgment under mild stress.

The primary value in the four-option drill is to get students to think outside of their own comfort zones.

Everyone has a fighting (or sparring or training) personality.[1] In the one-step, many default to striking, primarily hand striking. Four-option helps them get over this and look for new options.

---

[1] Training, sparring, fighting, or survival: You only know your personality at the level you have played. The next level up may be a complete surprise. Just as a diligent, hardworking student may be a powder puff the first time point sparring, a good point sparrer may well choke when the stakes rise to full contact . . . and a full-contact fighter frequently freezes under assault.

Do this: the four-option drill. Person A starts a technique and freezes. Person B then takes the time to evaluate the position and momentum and chooses four options—one to move or unbalance the threat, one to cause pain, one to cause damage, and one to shut down the person entirely. Just like in the formal one-step, each of these must be accomplished with a single motion. Preferably while simultaneously defending self and bettering position.

After demonstrating all four, person B chooses and executes one of them and freezes. Person A then evaluates, demonstrates all four, and chooses one to execute. Repeat.

[Redacted]: The Baby Drill

Specifics of drill redacted

I want you to know it is here, in case you hear about it, but the baby drill doesn't belong in a manual. If you read about it, you will think you know it and you can memorize what to do. It is one of those things you have to feel without warning.

See section T, "Tricks and One-Offs," for more information on drills that are useful only once.

Slow Man Drills OS3

People speed up on the one-step. It's natural. Humans want to "win" even if that concept has little place in skill building. It is significantly easier to "win" if your opponent is going in slow motion and you are going at normal speed. Amazing how that works.

Sometimes telling them to slow down or having them press on each other's eyes to show how slow they need to go works. Sometimes not. Frequently I explain that whenever possible you should do this drill slower than your opponent because that forces you to be efficient. Most get that.

There are two drills, the slow man stuff, that I use to emphasize the point. Part of it comes in the "sell" when you explain to the student why he is doing the drill. Again, if you are going slower than the other person, you must be more efficient or you will fail.

Do this: in the first variation, one of the partners gets two moves at a time and the other gets only one.

In the second, the one-step is fought as a two-on-one fight. A fourth person does the count. "One" and all three get one action. "Two" and all get another action from whatever position they are now in. "Three" and so on.

You will see a big increase in tactical thinking under this drill and, with the usual advantage of slow motion, they will have time to think of options they can test at speed later.

Three-Way Coaching

Everyone sees different things in the same situation. The more possibilities you see in a fight, the more options you have. In truth, in training, we rarely see what is right in front of us. We see what we have been trained to see. This means we also miss what we have subconsciously trained to miss.

Three-way coaching is a way to get different eyes from different backgrounds to share information. It requires students with a mix of backgrounds. Sometimes in a seminar format you can get close to a perfect mix. Sometimes not. I encourage you, for your own training, to look for partners with a wide diversity of backgrounds. (See Interlude #5: "The Violence-Prone Play Group.")

Do this: to set up three-way coaching, divide your class into three different groups. Ideally, one group will be students who are primarily strikers, another primarily grapplers and throwers, and a third group who consider themselves "street oriented" (e.g., cops grounded in defensive tactics, or reality-based self-defense students). You can substitute weapon-oriented fighters for one of the groups.

The exact mix of students in the class is not important. What is important is that when you break them up into groups of three, each group has three people who do not see things the same way.

In each group of three, two will begin the one-step and the third will coach using stop-action critique:

"Freeze. Go back one move. What about . . . ?"

Each member of the group will rotate through the coaching position. Only the coach is allowed to stop the drill and offer suggestions. At the end of the drill, each group will have some exposure to how different stylists think and see.

Within a style, you can do a variation by assigning a beginner, an intermediate practitioner, and a senior to each group.

Dance Floor Melee OS5

This requires a group, preferably at least twenty people who are proficient in the one-step. Proficiency means they can do it safely without constant supervision and keep to slow motion.

Do this: get them all to a small area—a specific section of floor or mat or, if you are training in a gym, the basketball key works well. Tell them that they happen to be on a crowded dance floor when a wild brawl breaks out. You will be doing the count. As you say each number, everyone gets one simultaneous action.

Part of the purpose of this drill is that it is fun. The students should be thinking tactically, using space and momentum more than technique.

Ideally, they should also be fighting toward a goal. Notice that you never tell them to stay and fight, but most do. It becomes another example of bringing subconscious rules and preconceptions into a situation.

It is also fun to introduce a weapon into the scenario. Just reach in and hand someone a training knife or a foam brick or padded stick as a stand-in for a broken pool cue. It will not change the dynamic that much, but after the debriefing, ask who noticed there was a weapon. Many won't. The ability to observe, to see, is critical in any chaotic situation. Your ability to respond to any danger is limited by the options and the hazards you see.

When a weapon is introduced, you can see how students get caught in the trap of seeing self-defense as a purely physical skill. Those who even notice the weapon (a minority) will still attempt to engage instead of leave and very few, if any, will try nonphysical solutions. Not even things as simple as warning others: "Knife! He's got a knife!"

Frisk Fighting

OS

Many people carry weapons, whether a gun or just a pocketknife. Frisk fighting can be played for fun or at a very serious level. At the serious level, each person should have training equivalents for what he carries every day. (I know one civilian who carries two guns, three knives, and a can of pepper spray.) Participants should wear the safe training equivalents exactly where they carry in real life.

Do this: at the fun level, everyone just picks up whatever training weapons are lying around and puts them anywhere, but not in hand.

Frisk fighting is a variation on the one-step but with this rule in place: you can use anything you find except what you brought to the game.

If you can do it in one motion, you can draw your opponent's gun or knife, but you cannot draw your own. It's very rare, but sometimes a really creative fighter will draw a weapon from someone else in the room, not his opponent. That kind of creativity should be encouraged.

Frisk fighting works a bunch of related skills and concepts.

- It makes people stay alert for opportunities.

- It forces people who carry weapons to consider and practice weapon retention.

- It gives an introduction—a very mild one—to fighting in an armed world.

- It rewards an educated touch sense—sometimes you feel the weapon before you see it.

- It becomes a component of, and an introduction to, environmental fighting.

Frisk fighting and environmental fighting are the reasons why no live weapons are allowed in the training area. No exceptions.

Environmental Fighting   OS7

This should only be included after people have been exposed to frisk fighting (OS6), dynamic fighting (D1), wall fighting (D3), and the ground movement series (GM1–6).

Do this: environmental fighting is simply the one-step drill with all the environmental factors in play. You can pick up and use found or improvised weapons. You can push or throw your opponent into a wall or corner. Bend him over a desk or make him trip over a curb. Rolling, you can and should pound his head into the mat (simulated pavement) and use a brick or access a weapon if possible.

Fighting in the real world happens in places. Cluttered places and messy places and slippery places. Places with stuff to trip over and hard corners and rocks and sticks and car antennas and garbage. Sometimes on floors littered with used syringes. Life sucks way worse in the real world than in a clean dojo that doesn't stink like alcohol sweat and meth and fear.

You can't safely play with syringes and blood exposures and disease. But you can go slow and play safely with the rest.

Again, the biggest aspect of self-defense is learning to see. It is better to see the situation coming and avoid it, but if not, you need to see opportunities. Opportunities to escape and opportunities to do damage.

Without practice, using the environment is a mystery to most martial artists. The trouble with not practicing seeing is that anything invisible to you can be used against you. In a fight the only difference between a hazard and a gift is who sees and exploits it first.

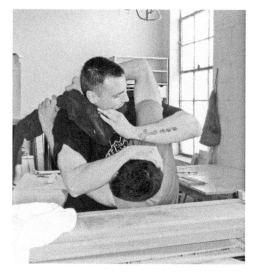
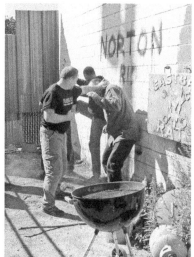
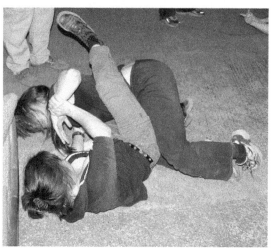
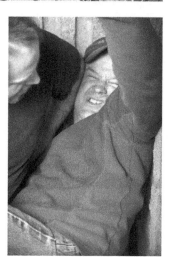

Environmental Fighting Situations.

The Brawl OS8

This is the culmination of the one-step.

It is done as a one-step for safety. With skill, the one-step gets very fast though. Doesn't matter as long as everyone goes at the same speed and can be safe. Everything is in play. We do this in a cluttered room (nightclubs, bars, and abandoned warehouses are my preference) with safe training weapons and frisk-fighting rules in effect.

Do this: the game is played with everyone against everyone and temporary alliances, using the environment and anything the fertile imaginations of the students come up with is allowed. The first time I introduced this drill with the tactical team, we played in extremely low-light conditions. It was a very good day.

When you are less certain about the group's proficiency and safety, you can conduct the brawl under the rules of the dance floor melee (OS6). Have one designated safety officer who keeps the time. The safety officer counts loudly and all participants simultaneously get a single move with each number counted.

INTERLUDE #1:
BIASES AND ASSUMPTIONS

Every instructor has biases and assumptions built into all aspects of training. I have them. So does your instructor. We can't help it. We see the world a certain way and certain things have worked for us. The things that worked (for us, in our environment) are where we concentrate our teaching.

An athletic martial artist who has worked as a bouncer will believe and teach that you see attacks coming and your physical attributes are key.

An instructor who has survived a rape attempt may well believe the key is unbridled ferocity—"slipping the leash." If she won despite disadvantages in strength, size, and position, she will believe and teach that strength, size, and position are secondary to mind-set. If she could not even think of a technique in the moment, she will likely teach that technique is irrelevant.

So here are my biases and assumptions, to the extent that I see them. The thing with blind spots is that you can't see them, so there are many I will miss.

- Unarmed arts only exist for emergencies you didn't see coming. If you can predict it and plan it and force is unavoidable, it is stupid to go in without a weapon. For that matter, without getting every advantage you can.

- Which means the basic environment of an unarmed encounter is the position of disadvantage. Bad structure, positioning, footing, injured, overwhelmed, and behind the curve.

- Almost always, the ones you see coming you can ward off by positioning or verbal de-escalation. As such, I've often—and (so far) successfully—put myself in positions that weren't tactically optimal in order to talk stuff down, which is strategically preferable.

- I don't think conflict is a physical problem most of the time (see above), and even when it is a physical problem, there are minds and social rules and the world involved. The more of those elements you can manipulate skillfully, the better off you are. Sometimes you play the cards, sometimes you play the person, and sometimes you play the table.

- I expect the threat to have the advantage in size and strength or to be crazy (mental instability or drugs). Because, in my experience, almost all of them were one or the other. Potentially a sampling error . . . but I think it makes sense, since you'd have to be crazy to routinely attack bigger and stronger people.

- I believe in the primacy of infighting, close-range combat. This is the prejudice that is most likely to be incompatible with a student's nature. Classical jujutsu is an infighting system—weapons were assumed and there was no safe way to finish it at long range. Early I learned that people freak out more when someone tries to close, and that shaped my personality. Thus, by nature and training, I'm an infighter. I tend to reject techniques that keep distance, and most of the techniques I prefer (and therefore teach) put you at clinch range. If that's not a good range for you, I'm unlikely to be a good teacher for you.

- I tend not to injure people. In corrections, the preferred outcome on my job was maximum control with minimum injury. That's shaped a lot in that I have very few strikes I consider reliable. Marc MacYoung, my friend and fellow trainer, consistently gives me a bad time because I don't always treat potentially deadly threats as seriously as he thinks I should.

- Weapons: I'm completely cool with improvised weapons and using obstacles. But for the first ten years of my career, we were not allowed to carry anything. When OC (pepper spray) was finally authorized, I just never thought about it. I would forget I was carrying spray. On the other hand, my weapon training was completely offensive, centered on hostage rescue tactics with a team. My mind-set is completely different when I pack versus when I don't.

- I have very weak social instincts. This means that I don't tend to get emotional or competitive when I fight . . . and I don't really understand why other people do. It's good in that the lack of anger never makes me want to overstep bounds, but some of my basic things—the range, positioning, not bothering to make eye contact, smelling, face contact—are sometimes hard for others. Many people have to force themselves to grab a face, for instance, whereas grabbing a collar or neck is (emotionally) easier. Just rarely as effective.

There are more, I'm sure. Do this analysis for yourself, your style, and your instructor. It all adds up to this: each of us is training for a generally narrow range of conflict. Including me. Be aware.

BLINDFOLD DRILLS

Safety issues with blindfolded training:

- As with all training, no live weapons in the training area.

- One person in each group must be able to see to prevent the blindfolded one(s) from running into one another or dangerous obstacles.

- Blindfolded people must go especially slowly. The standard for one-step drills is slowly enough that one can press directly on the eye.

Blindfolded Defense

This is done as a partner drill, and it begins with one partner blind-folded in a clinch position. There is a progression to the skill.

Do this: the unblindfolded partner initiates a slow, powerful attack. The blindfolded partner names the attack (e.g., "uppercut" or "low kick"). The attacks at first may be slow and slightly exaggerated. That's fine. Most people pick this up quickly, but some don't. The partner feeding the attacks should not try to be tricky. It is also more realistic. In an assault, the bad guy is trying to hurt you, not to trick. He will do his best to generate a lot of power.

In the next evolution, the attacks come faster, and the blindfolded partner just blocks them. It is actually easier than the first drill because the action/action dynamic bypasses the talking part of the brain. Most people feel the motion and flinch to a good blocking position.

If it is easier, works better, and is more applicable, why do we do the first evolution? Good question. I'm glad you asked. People are smart, and some will learn that they can sweep wide areas and "block" most attacks. If people are successful enough with slop, they tend to bypass core skills. The core skill here is sensitivity—precisely reading position and motion through contact.

The third evolution is to increase distance and decrease points of contact. Working from the clinch, the blindfolded partner has a lot of information. Stretch the arms out until each partner only has one hand in contact. Then play with the blindfolded player having one hand on the threat and no other points of contact.

Blindfolded work is much easier than most people believe. If you haven't done it, it may seem challenging or mystical. Once you have done it, it is simple and obvious.

As humans, we are all very similar: meat over bones. My bones are connected—leg to pelvis to spine to shoulder—just like yours. Once you have two points of contact (or one, with skill), you will feel any shift in my motion transmitted through the bones.

I have met a very few who have trained isolation to the extent that they can mask this movement. It's possible, but it is rare.

Coaching Blindfolded Defense:

- Emphasize repeatedly that this is a sensitivity drill, not a fighting exercise. If winning and losing get into the students' heads, they will tense up, speed up, and lose the benefits of the drill.

- People who are insensitive will try to sweep through likely area with a big motion. After all, if you just stretch your arm and make a big circle with it, it should block *something*. It's not necessary on this drill, and it allows them to have some success without getting the skill. If someone starts sweeping or guessing, pull him back to the first evolution of naming the incoming attack.

- You can do blindfolded drills with both partners blindfolded when they get a little experienced, but in a cluttered or even mildly crowded training area, one person should be tasked as a safety officer to make sure the blindfolded person doesn't fall into another group or the wall or something.

The first, obvious benefit of blindfolded drilling is that it is fun. Most students will have a big "gee whiz" moment when they realize they can actually do this.

It is a sensitivity drill, but you have to analyze exactly what sensitivity means in a given context. Just saying something is a sensitivity drill is a nonanswer.

The student learns to feel incoming forces. This is particularly important for a few reasons. One is that feeling force is far more accurate than trying to see force. Power coming in (for that matter, mass moving in any direction) can be exploited. When you feel it, you know immediately how much power and which direction. When you see it, you see the gross action of the body, the small action of the hands, shoulder and hip alignment, and foot position. Correlating all that takes too long to be useful most of the time.

It is quite common not to be able to see in a fight. Darkness, the threat behind you, and blood in your eyes come immediately to mind, but sometimes the action is so close—in your face—and so fast, with a flurry of strikes coming in, that the eyes can't handle it. Touch still can.

Touch also gives a faster reaction than focused sight and is less hampered by adrenaline. The cascade of stress hormones that accompanies a sudden assault frequently results in tunnel vision—you may see the scar on the ring finger of the fist coming at your face but be completely incapable of seeing the threat's feet, other hand, or face.

Reaction time to touch is faster than peripheral vision reaction time and much faster than focused vision, so blindfolded work can make you faster in infighting.

And now for the cool effect. Touch is not just faster than sight. As you develop skill, you will find yourself responding not to the incoming attack, but to the precursors. Most people shift their center of gravity slightly to chamber or set up a strike or kick. Any motion, really. For example, before you take a step forward, you lean slightly back to put your center of gravity over the foot you aren't moving. The shift happens before the motion.

Between the reaction speed of touch and the fact that you act on precursor movements, you will find yourself defending actions before they happen, sometimes before the threat has consciously decided to move. You can almost call it combat precognition.

Blindfolded Targeting

When I demonstrate this at seminars, I pick someone from the crowd, blindfold her, and walk up behind. At full arm extension I slap my hand down on her shoulder and say, "Slowly, so that you don't break anything, kick my lead knee." Over 80 percent of the time, with no training or practice, the kick is dead on.

Then I leave my hand where it is and shift my body to one side or the other and give the same instruction. Most of the time the kick is accurate. Despite the hand in the same place, the difference in tension in the fingers is enough for a blindfolded person to know exactly where my knee is. Without ever having done it before!

Do this: start from the clinch again and the unblindfolded partner names targets—floating ribs, throat, ear, back knee—and the blindfolded partner touches the target slowly and with an appropriate weapon (kick, knee, fist, elbow, slap).

Almost everyone gets the blindfolded defense right away. This is harder. Remind the students to feel, not think, and if they miss, to just

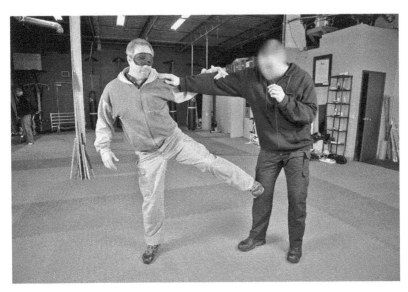

Blindfolded knee kick

find the target. Make it precise. An inch off the solar plexus is a miss. Find the precise target; then do it again.

As they get better, distance can be increased and points of contact decreased, just like in the last drill.

It is important to go slowly for safety.

Core Fighting

This doesn't need to be done blindfolded, but it often helps.

As mentioned before, the body is made of bone wrapped in meat. That means every part of you is connected. If I push your shoulders, I can affect your hips and legs. The shoulder girdle is a big lever arm attached to the pelvis, and the pelvis is a lever arm as well.

It's a subtle skill in a real fight, but I have used it effectively to avoid more damaging options.

Do this: have one partner (A) put her hands on B's shoulders. When B lifts his left leg to kick, A pulls out and down with her right hand on B's left shoulder. He has to put his foot back on the ground to maintain his balance. The kick is aborted.

This is a drill that must be played with, not performed in rote steps. Motion in one direction puts the foot back on the ground. Motion in the other direction, however, can tweak the balance so badly that the person can't kick with any power. Pushing, pulling, twisting, and all the variations and combinations have some effect, and the students need to play with them to see what is possible and, most importantly, to get the feel for what the threat is about to do.

I've overheard some students affectionately refer to this drill as puppet-mastering. That's appropriate.

There are two related concerns with this drill. The first is that if it is introduced too soon, the students will not develop the sensitivity described in the other versions. That is why this is the last simple blindfold drill taught. The second concern is similar: just keeping constant stress—pushing, pulling, and jerking in random directions—is extremely effective . . . and so if you puppet-master too aggressively too early, it is a very effective skill. Like many very effective tricks, students tend to miss what makes them work, which, again, is sensitivity.

Blindfolded Infighting

Depending on your confidence in the students, their control and skill, and your normal rules and tolerances for contact, there are different ways this can be played.

Do this: you can work from the one-step drill with one or both partners blindfolded. Whenever you play with two blindfolded people, you need a third person acting as a safety monitor. Running into walls or other people can be bad.

I strongly suggest you start this drill at close quarters with one person attacking from the rear or the flank.

If your students are ready, I sometimes do close-quarters sparring. Again, starting back to chest or chest to side (the aggressor in the dominant position starts the action). This is sparring and will depend on your sparring rules. In the dojo where I trained jujutsu, it was no holds barred and light to stiff contact. (I cannot imagine doing full contact and no holds barred with anyone I respected without a fatality or crippling injury.) That means that strikes (including kicks, elbows, knees, and headbutts), locks, throws, gouges, spine manipulations, and grappling were all on the table. And biting.

Blindfolds really didn't change the game that much. If you've been sparring like that for any length of time, you don't rely on your eyes very much anyway.

Whether you do this as blindfolded one-step or blindfolded sparring, it's a good time.

One thing your students will learn: if you lose contact with your opponent, you're screwed. This drill really reinforces the primacy of infighting. If you don't teach the primacy of infighting (as all right-thinking people do), you may want to skip this drill.

An e-mail from an old student telling me about his twelve-year-old daughter:

I've been messing around with Allie for a couple years now. A while back we played with dead hands just so she'd know you didn't need to make a fist to thump someone. We talked about the concept, she thumped on me a bit, I thumped on her (gently!), and didn't think anything more of it. On Monday evening we were cleaning up the kitchen, and I started harassing her (like I always do). And she thumped me. Right on the left joint of my mandible. With a perfect dead hand. (I could feel where the heel of her hand hit me, and the tips of three of her fingers.)

This was interesting for a number of reasons:

1. Good god that hurt like HELL. I have TMJ so I'm no stranger to pain in that joint, but that was a new and radical form. Sweet.

2. My eyes rolled up in my head and everything went red/black. That was cool. Total disconnect from my body. There were two things in the world—the joint (which felt like it had exploded), and my left hand, which was resting on Allie's right shoulder. And you know what? Just through that one point of contact on her I had a perfect wireframe (it was red) in my head of how she was positioned. I saw EVERYTHING—her shoulder angle, arm positions, hip angle, and leg positions (but not her feet. It didn't extend below her knees) through that one point of contact. That was SO FRIGGIN' COOL. All the blind fighting we did with T-shirts wrapped around our heads taught me something. Heh.

    The only thing I don't know is if I closed my eyes in reaction to the pain in my jaw hinge or if she really did shut me down.

3. My daughter can inflict that much pain with one hand. My 12-year-old daughter (100 pounds wringing wet) can do THAT. Muahahahahahahaha!

4. The scary bit was immediately running through a bunch of responses to the situation. I discarded the first 10 (I had no idea I knew so many ways to hurt people—thank you) and just wrapped my arms around her in a big hug. That was definitely a cool experience—I'd like to try that again in a controlled environment just to make sure I do have as good a control over myself as I thought I did, but I don't know how to do that without doing permanent damage to my jaw hinge. Darned thing still hurts. Heh.

    Anyway, that was cool beyond words. Thought I'd share.

D: DYNAMIC FIGHTING

Every time I see a self-defense instructor teach an escape from a bear hug, it puzzles me. The only people I ever see bear hug and just stand there are cops and bouncers—the good guys. For most, a bear hug grip is something you use to slam someone into a wall or throw someone into a closet or car trunk. It is fast and mobile: you are whipped off your feet.

Most of the defenses taught don't work so well when you are swinging through the air.

Fighting is dynamic. It happens moving. Even with firearms and the emphasis on the range with a stable platform and good sight picture . . . gunfights involve a lot of running and ducking.

If you have practiced either static defenses or the largely two-dimensional motion of sparring, the wild action of a fight will be unfamiliar. The crashing, running, pushing, pulling, and dropping can confuse you. Worse, if your skills require a solid base, they will simply fail.

At the same time, if you use it, the energy in a dynamic system is a gift. Every push, pull, and even strike is something you can use. If you know how.

Dynamic Fighting

This drill is best done with gi jackets or other heavy shirts. Like most skills, you can do them on T-shirts or bare skin, but you don't often get attacked by naked people, and whereas a good gi will last a year, you'll destroy a couple of T-shirts a night.

There are two distinct roles in the drill:

Do this: one person is assigned as the manipulator. He or she pulls and pushes the other around like a rag doll. The goal is not merely to muscle but to find more efficient ways to push and pull a person and disrupt a threat's balance. The participants will find, for instance, that curling the little finger in has great unexpected force, that dropping weight down and backward is nearly irresistible, and that pushing or pulling with an upward vector or a spiral is more effective than doing so with a horizontal action.

The manipulator plays with all of these things with an eye to owning the skills, making pushing someone around second nature.

The user's role is to find the gift, to find the precise moment where the manipulator's force can be exploited and a slight action can take the manipulator off balance and, ideally, plant him into a wall.

If you have played in judo, classical jujutsu, or wrestling, this concept will be very familiar. If you have played American football or rugby and practiced spinning out of a tackle, you have a good piece of it. If you have practiced aikido, the concept will be second nature, but you may have to adjust to the hands-on physicality of it.

If you have mats and the students are skilled at breakfalls, this is a perfect drill for perfecting the *sutemi waza* (sacrifice throws) and to some extent the *makikomi waza* (winding throws). These throws are particularly effective when there is a great disparity in strength or force between a strong attacker and a weak defender.

This drill should always be played with an eye toward using the environment. Within the bounds of safety, the user should try to get the manipulator to run into a wall or obstacle. That is the skill that can turn the natural chaos of a fight into your home field advantage.

Coaching points:

- To exploit the moment of weakness, most of the time the user merely needs to drop a shoulder when the manipulator pushes.

- There can be power in momentarily resisting and then collapsing your own structure. It can sucker the manipulator into adding more pressure.

- That said, the biggest problem, especially with young men, will be the need to dominate. They will go force against force to stop the manipulator, to prove they are the stronger male, and then try to apply technique . . . but stopping takes all of the momentum out of the system.

Sumo

Sumo, as it is often seen, is a big ritual played by enormous men. It is actually one of the best systems ever devised to train balance and exploiting momentum.

The rules are simple. Two people enter a ring. If either touches the ground with anything except the soles of his feet or touches the ground outside the ring, he loses.

Do this: as a training drill, I allow no strikes and no clothing grips. It will start as a contest of strength as the two players try to force each other out of the ring . . . until one suddenly reverses, pulling instead of pushing, and the other loses his balance.

The game is uniquely designed to showcase how little power it takes to redirect force and how much it takes to overwhelm it.

The Hole against the Wall   **D3**

Whenever you can, you should fight emptiness. That sounds absurdly mystical, but it isn't. If someone is facing you with his fists up, you don't want to fight where his fists are; you want to fight where they aren't. Like behind him.

It is so much easier to neutralize a threat from behind I am almost embarrassed to mention it . . . and yet I know very few nongrapplers who train in taking someone out from behind and even fewer who practice crossing to the rear. It is a skill.

Fighting emptiness is everywhere: many locks only work because people fight against the force. Most locks have a huge gap where the locked limb can just be pulled out . . . but the instinct to fight force is so strong that the easy way might as well be invisible.

The hole against the wall drill is a way of learning to see these empty zones in an unlikely place.

Do this: one person pins another up against a wall. It is irrelevant how the pin happens—double shoulder, across the throat, anything.

The person pinned takes a deep breath, if necessary, and feels the wall, the force from her opponent, and finds the hole. The hole is the place where she can slip or collapse or weasel and the threat will fall into the wall.

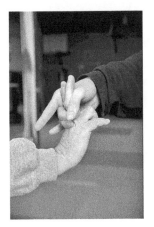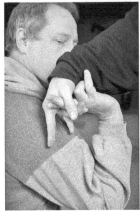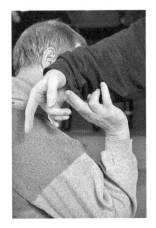

Holes in Locks

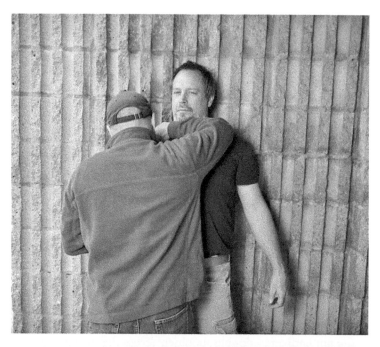

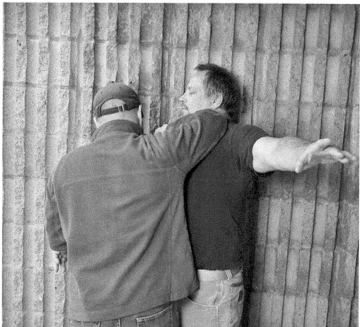

Arm sweep on wall escape.

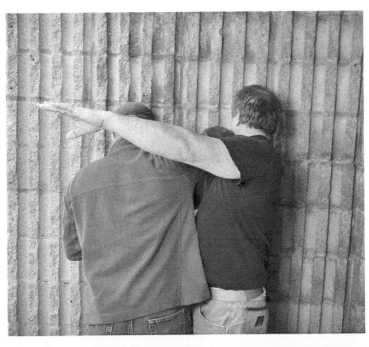

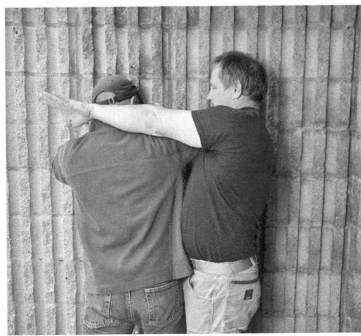

The physics are basic. If I am pinning you up against the wall, I am leaning on you, adding weight to the system. If I am leaning, I am off balance by definition. *You* are holding me up. You do not fight me; you merely cease to support me.

There are tactics that make this easier. Large arm sweeps on a plane parallel to your body applied against the leverage point in the threat's arm, for instance—or creating bubbles of space against the wall for you to collapse into.

This drill may require feeling and seeing to understand, but once it starts to work, it is obvious.

Coaching tip: a lot of people are going to want to push the threat away and use that added space for the threat to fall into. It works, provided you are strong enough to push the threat away in the first place. It is nearly always unnecessary, and unnecessary effort is wasted effort.

Moving in the Clinch

Do this: partners clinch up and just practice making each other move, paying attention to foot placement, center of gravity (CoG) and base, and applying power to weak lines. Notice that the two partners actually make a single unit with a four-point base and a shared CoG but that this can be changed by disengaging (allowing one party to lose balance if the move is clean enough) or even exploiting the shared momentum, as in a sutemi waza (sacrifice throw).

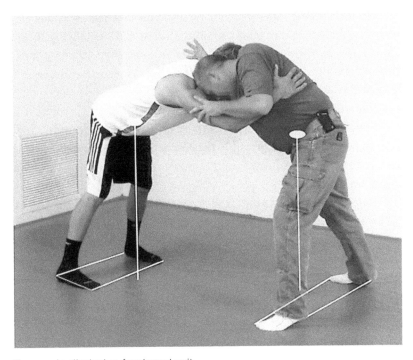

Two people clinched as four-legged unit

French Randori

About the name—I have no idea why it is called French randori. That's what it was called when I first learned it.

This is mostly for students who regularly practice throws and takedowns. It is not safe to practice any takedowns unless you have good breakfall skills and good mats (or excellent skills and poor mats).

Randori is the generic term for judo sparring (and sparring in other systems like jujutsu and aikido). Randori has two players going for throws and then on the ground going for strangles, arm locks, or pins.

Do this: French randori is for throws and takedowns. It has elements of the original dynamic fighting drill as well as moving in the clinch. The partners take turns, one manipulating the other pushing, pulling, and overbearing. The other waits for his chance and goes for a clean throw or takedown. Then they switch roles.

It is simply taking turns going for the throw.

French randori is another sensitivity drill. By taking turns the goal is to remove as much as possible the competitive element and learn to feel and see the mix of forces and opportunity that creates a throw in a real confrontation.

Remind the students that if they get too competitive, if they block all incoming throws, they don't get a turn.

INTERLUDE #2: SOURCES

Always be careful where you get your information. People, including you, love to have an outside authority validate what they already believe. That is a dangerous trap. You will learn far more from people who disagree with you than from people who tell you what you already believe.

As an instructor, student, or just functionally intelligent individual, there are two things you must do:

1. Evaluate sources.

2. Cultivate good sources.

Evaluating sources is not that hard. It is largely a matter of understanding your personal epistemology, being clear about what you know and what you do not know, and evaluating your own situation.

Epistemology is how you decide what is "true." Which sources you trust without thinking about it. Too many people assume that certain professions or certain histories imply some validity. Do cops know more about violence than civilians? Do soldiers know more than cops? Do elite officers (like SWAT) or elite soldiers know even more?

Sort of. And that's one of the keys. Anyone who deals with violence or bad guys professionally will know more than people who don't, but what they know may not apply to you.

Police officers have far more force options (weapons) than most civilians could ever carry. They have radios, backup, and, unless they screw up, the angels in dispatch know where they are and what they are doing. Further, they have a duty to act, which means that preclusion, one of the hallmarks of self-defense in most states, is not an issue. And, most of the time, they are the ones responding to a situation—they are going in with little time to evaluate, plan, gather resources, and possibly create surprise.

What about elite cops?

The whole point about being elite is to apply more training, equipment, skills, and higher-order teamwork to make extremely dangerous situations as safe as possible. I did some things with my team that, on paper, were mind-numbingly dangerous . . . but I always felt safe with my team.

Tactical teams are hunters, and they know what they are doing.

Detectives, another form of elite, rarely use force. Protocol in most agencies is for uniform backup if things might go bad. But the best detectives know criminals inside and out.

Soldiers? Experts at using offensive force to eliminate an enemy. They have rules of engagement, but self-defense is a legal concept that applies to civilians. Wartime is very different.

And elite soldiers . . . most get some time with unarmed self-defense skills, but true professionals are utterly pragmatic. Bullets beat punches.

So these professionals know violence, some at a level that makes it hard to sleep—enough dead to dam a river, not the executed or soldiers, but women raped and murdered in a certain civil war not so long ago—but it may not be the knowledge that you need.

Going in on an entry to a crack house is not the same skill you might need to deal with a home invasion or carjacking. Ambushing a convoy (or surviving a convoy ambush) has little to do with preventing a rapist from talking his way into your apartment.

There is no position or accolade that makes someone an automatic expert in what *you* might need. Learn what you can learn—some can help you stay cool under pressure; most have little lifesaving tricks and perspectives on awareness. Some know evil and how bad guys operate, and that is something you need to know.

For fairness, evaluate me: I'm a veteran corrections officer, former soldier (nothing special, medic assigned to a National Guard anti-armor infantry unit), and I spent fourteen months as an advisor in Iraq.

What does that mean? Working direct supervision, I've spent more waking hours with criminals than you want to know. I've listened in on conversations and read their private journals. Interviewed, interrogated, and even played chess with them.

Working booking, a corrections officer will have more uses of force in two years than the average enforcement officer will have in a career. And, unlike an enforcement officer, corrections works unarmed (though that is changing).

Sounds good, right? It doesn't mean as much as you think. I was in good shape, well trained, and knew the environment I was working in. I can teach about bad guys. A little about unarmed responses to ambushes and multiple opponents. About the weapon culture in the criminal subculture . . . Cool. But I have never been a 110-pound female targeted for an abduction rape. Never been caught in a cycle of domestic violence.

There is much I don't know. Much any instructor doesn't know. Be wary of any instructor who wants to sell you answers to your problems based on unrelated experiences.

Be clear about what you know and what you do not know. Truth is, you don't *know* very much. Do you *know* I'm a former corrections officer? Or do you think that because I said so? I don't know if YMAA has done a background check on me. My publishers may not be sure . . .

And it might not mean anything. People outside the cop world attach a lot of weight to things that make no sense to us. We have an expression, "training geek," for someone who goes into training full time with negligible street experience. It's not only possible; it's common. One local agency puts its burnouts in one particular division with a very elite designation so they can retire while looking good. I know one man who was promoted explicitly because he was not safe to work the streets.

You may not have the information to accurately judge an instructor's background. So what do you do? You pay attention to your common sense. Does the instructor make sense to *you*? Can *you* use what you are learning? Is the training about the instructor's ego or the student's progress?

Get this: I'm not fraud busting here. A guy who has spent ten years teaching other cops has done that, even if he has never been in a real fight himself. It doesn't invalidate the training. What I am saying is that your training is always about *you*. If you put your instructor on a pedestal because he wore a green beret or has a tenth-degree black belt, you have quit thinking for yourself. I'm not trying to bust the résumé or the rank; I'm trying to bust the pedestal, which *you* brought to the table and is turning off *your* brain.

Evaluating your own situation.

Most people live productive, stable, safe lives. Before you can evaluate a teaching's relevance, you have to take a good, hard look at the types of danger you are likely to face.

I am worried about prison-style shankings because most of the people who might have some reason to kill me use that technique. Never pissed off a convict? Not something you need to worry about.

One of the most dangerous types of attacks is a betrayal group monkey dance, where all available members of a group have a little violence party on your body. It is 100 percent avoidable with a two-step process: (1) Don't join a violent group, and (2) if you do join one, don't betray them.

So you need to work out your personal threat profile at some point (see WW11: "Personal Threat Assessment") and see what you are likely to face. Then compare it to the threat assessment of your instructor. A fit six-foot, shaved-headed martial arts instructor and bouncer will get a fair amount of violence, largely from drunk college kids who don't like being kicked out of bars. The opponents will likely be, well, drunk college kids.

Someone skilled at those problems may not be able to help someone whose threat profile centers on acquaintance rape or ambush assaults.

Cultivate good sources.

There are a million things you don't know. Ten million. Some ridiculously high number. Good. Same for me. Same for all of us.

Make friends and develop contacts with people who live in different worlds. My elite military friends don't necessarily know what I need, but I'll never give them up as friends or as advisors because I can never know what I'll need in the future. They know things I don't.

Keep friends in the cop world and the criminal world, the military world and the martial arts world. And keep some friends and contacts in the peaceful, friendly world as well, because that is who we do this for anyway.

My super-traditionalist martial friends know body mechanics and history in a way that my military friends never will . . . and the military guys look at terrain in a way that very few martial artists are ever taught. The cops know bad guys, and if we don't know the enemy, what are our chances?

But also get to know your students and get to know professionals who think clearly and can represent your students.

I'm a guy. Been one all my life. Because of that there are things I am profoundly ignorant about that are common knowledge to women. I had no idea, until recently, that almost all women for very good reason are fearful when there is a long hallway to the bathroom in a bar or restaurant. Or how hard it is to conceal a weapon under female business attire. Or the difficulties wasp-waisted women have in drawing from a standard hip holster.

If you are teaching women (or any group you are not a member of), you need to cultivate sources that can fill you in on problems. Then you need to be able to work solutions for their circumstances, not yours.

The average woman is smaller, weaker, and has less experience than the average violent criminal. One of my sources, a skilled martial artist, says she is routinely outweighed by 50–100 percent and the average guy has twice to three times her strength. How many guys could give up one hundred or two hundred pounds and the first move and still win? And if you can't, do you really have anything to teach for women's self-defense?

F: FUNDAMENTALS

This section will cover some things I consider basics. Some fundamentals are too basic to require specific drills. Power generation, for instance, has to be taught, and then you go apply it on a heavy bag (at first) and then an armored opponent. What follows are important things, some little, some major, that lend themselves well to simple exercises.

Maai with Weapons

Maai, the ability to accurately judge distance, is critical, especially in any form of armed combat. If something is going to miss, you don't waste energy or time defending . . . but it takes a well-trained and educated eye to judge finely when you will be missed.

Do this: this drill develops the skill over time. You can start without weapons. Like most drills, it is simple. You stand facing your opponent. You start by guessing.

Each limb has a different reach. The rear leg will have the longest reach, the rear hand the shortest. You will choose a personal weapon (rear hand, rear leg, lead hand, or lead leg) and stand as close as you can and still be out of range. Then let your partner strike.

Straight and circular strikes do not change the range. The bones are only so long and attached at either the shoulder or the pelvis. Leaning does change range, but a slight slip or lean away at a slight angle often is enough to compensate for a lean.

Practice this stage with as many different partners and different body types as possible until it is instinctive. The goal is to practice until you know a strike will miss, and so you do not flinch away. People not only flinch, but they even block techniques that are going to miss anyway. Not only does that waste time and effort, but it slows down your own ability to close and attack, especially if you have to recover from your own defensive action.

In practicing the drill you will probably discover "ghosting." If your shoulders are slightly ahead of your hips, most people will misread you as being closer than you are. You can present an image, a ghost, of being in range for the rear-leg kick when in fact you are slightly out of range. It also makes your other targets seem easy to hit when your body's natural (and therefore fast) reaction will pull them out of range in plenty of time.

Practice both setting up and reading stances that confuse range—leans, shifting a heel slightly forward, and shoulder sets. Crossing feet can confuse range, but the best reaction is simply to knock a person with crossed feet on his ass. (First rule: No matter how cool, don't practice things that will get you killed.)

If you misjudge distance by a fraction of an inch and get hit . . . so what? The penetration, and therefore the damage, is negligible. It stings a bit. That's part of life.

This is also why practicing this unarmed is good for coordination development and has some advantage for sparring—but is almost useless for surviving assaults or real fighting. Experienced bad guys do not duel and do not play at the critical-distance line. They attack from ambush or talk their way well into the optimum range and then unleash a flurry of damage. Unarmed combat is not a matter of millimeters.

Armed fights sometimes are.

When you are ready, you graduate to weapons. The basics are the same, but now you must, with a glance, take in the length of the weapon and the grip.

If there is one reason to study sword in the modern era, it is because it ingrains an instinctive appreciation of maai like nothing else. I can't officially recommend doing this drill with live steel, but you damn sure learn fast that way.

Practice with long and short sword, ax, spear, staff, stick . . . anything and everything you can find. You have to read stance, just like before, but now grip: which hand limits the range? If it is a two-handed grip, the rear hand usually limits the range, but if he crosses up on the grip, he is preparing to shift to a single lead hand, which will add over a foot of range . . .

On a shafted weapon, like a spear, is one hand set to slide, like a pool cue? Again, the rear hand almost always controls the distance, unless the person is willing to risk losing his grip.

With weapons, crossing feet is sometimes practical because of the range difference. Where is the natural direction to uncoil?

So you practice the following:

1. finding the line where you will just barely be missed;
2. reading the angle in a slash (sometimes it is three dimensional and instead of moving back or angling, you just need to duck or duck and angle slightly);
3. ghosting range;

4. stepping barely into range and leaning out to coil the rear leg for a launch; and

5. recognizing when you are too far in range to escape and closing ruthlessly.

Off-Lining

Backing up is almost never the answer. Unless you are excellent at reading and remembering tactical terrain, you might not know what or who is behind you. You probably wouldn't be falling back if you were winning anyway, and falling back keeps you in the threat's sight. Last, you can't run backward as fast as a bad guy can run forward. Going straight back is almost always a losing battle.

Tactically, it is just easier to take someone down (or get away) from behind or the flank. This is one of the places where good tactics, otherwise known as intelligence, goes up against social conditioning, sometimes called stupid dominance games.

When fighting humans, humans want to fight eye to eye. They want the other person to see the face of the person who won and acknowledge dominance. This is so ingrained that even people who know better and who have trained specifically to get behind wind up standing toe to toe, throwing wild punches, and eventually rolling around on the ground.

Off-lining is not a new idea. The concept is inherent in karate kata. Aikido has dozens of techniques to get there. Rear naked strangle is the perfect position in grappling systems . . .

Get this: as socialized humans, we fight other humans. We play dominance games. A serious criminal is past that. He has already dehumanized you to the point that he can use violence. He doesn't need to work himself up to fight and for that matter, won't fight at all. He takes you out.

Think about it. You don't need to work yourself up or turn it into a contest or "fight" any animal that you kill for food or any flies that you swat or mice that you trap. The human predator is thinking of you this way, as a resource. It allows him to use extreme force very quickly, something most humans can't do. You will not beat a predator by playing a dominance game.

So for at least two reasons—because playing in the threat's target zone is stupid and to get to a better position—we need to practice getting off the line.

Fast off-lining involves the drop step. The drop step is inherent in all striking arts (though rarely explained) and was best described in Jack Dempsey's long-out-of-print book *Championship Fighting: Explosive Punching and Aggressive Defense.*

The drop step is deliberately falling. It uses gravity as a speed and power multiplier, and gravity doesn't telegraph. There are no tells to falling.

Do this: stand with your feet shoulder width or a little more apart and suddenly lift one. You will immediately begin falling to that side— if you do it right, which you won't at first.

Trained martial artists have been told since the first day to always stay on balance. Now some schmoe is writing in a book that some- times it is very useful to fall on purpose. So you go with your years of training and subtly, subconsciously, shift your weight to your left foot before raising your right. So you don't fall right away, but slowly, like a teetering tree. Furthermore, the shift of weight to the other side is the telegraph that the technique shouldn't have.

If your right foot snaps up with no attempt to control balance, you will move, falling faster than you could step.

Often, saying the words doesn't help. The trick I use is to snap my right foot to touch my left knee as quickly as I can. The effect you want is not a step, but like a leg has suddenly been removed from a stool.

Your foot will get back to the ground in time to keep you from falling down.

One of the fastest ways to learn the drop step is by having your partner throw straight punches at the center of your face. He knows you are moving, so he has to guard against anticipating or tracking your movement. If necessary, make him shut his eyes when he punches. You simply fall to the side.

Start slow with the punches. As the fall becomes more reflexive, it will work against faster and faster punches. There is a limit, of course. You begin the fall on seeing the punch, so it won't beat the action/reaction gap, but neither will a block or slip if the strike isn't telegraphed.

When that is comfortable at decent speed, start angling, using the drop step to fall at forty-five degrees toward the threat. You will find you don't need to change your foot position. Your back leg can launch you without slowing the fall (and here we replicate the body mechanics of the fencer's lunge).

Because you are not falling directly out of line, you may want a little insurance. If you are falling forward left, your left foot will be lifted. Bring your left hand up in a natural circle so it crosses your face and ends with the back of your left hand almost touching your right ear.

If your drop step is perfect, you won't need the insurance. If not, the circle will gently intercept the hand and glide it. Often, the partner

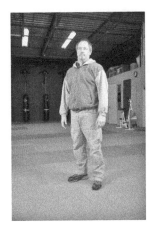
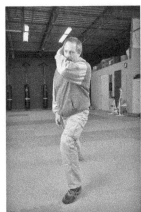
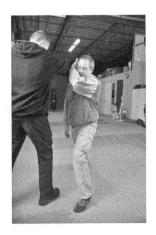
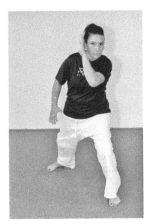
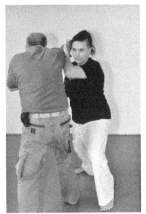

Drop step + mirror block

will not even know he missed. Do *not* try to aim the block or intercept the punch or push on the arm. Just make the circle and let physics take care of the rest.

Coaching point: For some reason, people like to use the rear hand with the lead leg. Watch for it. It doesn't work in this motion.

The last piece is recovery. Your partner punches, you drop step off line, paying the insurance, and then you pivot toward him, bringing your rear leg under you for a solid base. You've now flanked him and successfully evaded the attack. He is your cat toy.

If he was giving you a lot of reach, like a karate lunge punch, you will actually be behind him. If he is going full speed and you drop step and pivot, it has the interesting effect, from his point of view, of you getting behind twice as fast as a human can move. Nice.

Note: the drop step is also a great power multiplier. Once you have it down, practice falling into your strikes. Use it to close distance and strike for entries, to make your punches and short-range elbows more efficient. A drop step to the rear or rear flank using the point of the elbow as a spear can even injure someone behind you.

Targeting

Hitting requires power, timing, and a good target. Hitting a big bone with a little bone is more likely to damage your fist than a skull. The upper chest can take a huge amount of force without impairing function.

All hard-won lessons.

Targets have to be learned and they have to be practiced.

Do this: the targeting drill is simple. One partner stands like a statue in any position. The other partner works all the way around the statue's body, 360 or 720 degrees, launching a light-contact attack at all the targets he or she can think of. Work it like a continuous flow of constant damage and have fun.

It's educational to watch as well. Beginners know very few targets, their footwork is awkward as they circle, and they don't play with range. Experienced martial artists do, but some (and this is stylistic) miss entire categories of attacks or targets. Some will work pressure points and others will ignore them. Some will unbalance, wrap, and lock. Others won't. Some will ignore the legs as targets.

You learn a lot from watching people with different training experimenting with any drill.

Lock Flow

Locks may not be a part of your training. If they aren't, feel free to skip this section.

Some people say that you can't use locks, particularly small-joint locks, in a real fight. I've done so extensively, and therefore I disagree. There are several reasons for this. Years of training, decisive movement, and, possibly most important, the fact that I'm not married to the idea. If I get a lock, swell. If I don't or miss one or lose one, I transition immediately to something else.

One of the most important distinctions is that I never go into a situation looking for a particular lock. Locks and throws, in my experience, are always gifts. The bad guy puts himself in a position where the lock or throw is just there and I finish it for him.

In order to do the lock flow drill, you must be thoroughly familiar with joint locks. It will work if you have memorized a bunch of locks for all the major joints, but it will flow easier if you understand what locks are and the common principles.

Locks rely on gifts. You will not get an elbow lock on someone pulling in, but that action will hand you a shoulder lock, a wristlock, or both. Pushing gives up the elbow . . . If you have played with joints enough, you will understand this instinctively.

The lock flow drill is conducted much like the one-step. It is slow and noncompetitive. The partners must communicate. Tapping is important, but just saying, "That's good" or "You need to rotate a little more to get it . . ." is critical. These are partners, not enemies.

Do this: partner A stands in any position. Partner B then applies a lock of any kind. It is not fast or hard and not meant to move A or hurt, just to demonstrate a lock. Partner A then flows out of the lock.

Flowing out can take some explanation. Most locking styles teach rolling or flowing with the force of the lock. That's one way. But a slight shift into or away from most locks can take the elbow, for instance, off the fulcrum point and the lock vanishes. Unless they are based out, locks have a big hole perpendicular to the line of force in the lock where there is absolutely nothing keeping the person from just pulling out, except for the instinct to fight against pressure instead of emptiness. Many locks have nothing to prevent a lateral rotation out of the lock.

Any of these methods is acceptable; just don't rely on strength. If you do use strength, use it smart. Instead of trying to muscle out of a wristlock, just grab the hand with your other hand and pull it to your chest. Works like magic, most of the time.

Once A has escaped from the lock, he examines B's position and finds the lock that B is giving him. If an arm is straight, there's an elbow lock. Elbow bent close to ninety degrees? Just a twist away from a shoulder lock. Extended finger or two? Sweet.

A takes the gift. B flows out and starts looking for a gift . . .

It is a continuous flow drill, far more about learning to see opportunities than applying technically perfect locks.

When coaching, remind the students that locks don't require hands all the time. There will be lots of opportunities to lock with waist, neck, shoulder . . . almost infinite possibilities.

Initiative

Decisive action, exploding without telegraphing, is a critical ability. It is important in sparring. It is even more important when someone has you cold, at gunpoint for instance, and you know you need to move.

Action beats reaction. If I move and you are keying on my motion, I will be on you before you have processed the fact that you are under attack. That's the way it is supposed to work, but relatively few people just move. They set up first. They *prepare* to move. It is totally unnecessary and costs them the advantage.

Do this: the drill is simple. With my arm fully extended, I hold a training knife at your throat. You do something. That's it.

With the arm fully extended, I'm not much of a threat. There's little I can do. You do not want this drill to turn into a speed contest or have the person with the knife trying to manipulate the unarmed one by feinting or twitching.

The unarmed person does something, and this is the key. Almost anything works. You can slap the hand away. You can trap and close. You can even lean away and kick . . . all provided there is no telegraph.

If the person with the knife sees or senses any motion whatsoever, he slashes the weapon down the chest.

If you hold the knife, you will see the student tense, or look at what he plans to attack or take a deep breath, sometimes all of these, and then the shoulder drops and the hand comes back before it goes forward . . . there is usually plenty of time, at first.

Not one of these actions is necessary. Not breathing, not retraction, not focusing the eyes. Not one of those precursors makes the action faster or stronger. Just more predictable.

The person telegraphs, you drag the knife down his chest, and tell him what you saw. Repeat.

The skill is not in the motion but in practicing the stillness.

Stillness can spread to other areas of your life. People have serious trouble reading people who wait in stillness. Most find it spooky, especially in a bad situation where everyone is panicked or at least excited and one person is simply still. And the still one will act first, and decisively, when it is time to act.

Eventually, this should spread to all of your techniques. Just move. Don't think about it or set or prepare. Just move. Just cut. Just strike. Just close.

Advanced Ukemi

Ukemi, the art of falling without getting hurt, is a critical skill. Takedowns at some level are a natural part of the fight, and many people get hurt on impact. You must get skilled at falling. If you don't currently train breakfalls, find someplace where you can learn.

Realistically, only a very small percentage of martial arts students will ever use their skills to defend themselves from attack. Most, if not all of them, will fall down at some point. Knocked down, slip on ice, trip . . . doesn't matter. In protection from probable injury, breakfalls are the most important skill in the entire martial arts repertoire.

Advanced ukemi are a set of skills and games that get you used to flying through the air while evaluating your landing zones. Most are based on rolling falls and dive rolls, but you also have to have flat falls down cold. In a fight, the thrower, not the throwee, chooses the type of breakfall. If you only train rollouts because they are so much more efficient and the bad guy simply hangs on so that you can't roll, you will hit hard.

Do these:

- Wall rolls. This is an evasion technique. You run full speed directly at a wall. As you close, you spear one arm diagonally across your body so the hand hits the wall and you "roll" down the arm. This will spin you fast, 270 degrees to the side, now parallel to the wall, still on your feet and still running.

- Pick up. Scatter training weapons across the training floor. Dive roll and pick up the weapon as you land. Try to secure the weapon while you are in the air and before you roll. Have the weapon in hand and ready when you roll to your feet.

- Draw. Draw a weapon while falling and rolling. This is hard, and sword scabbards get in your way. Drawing a weapon without a scabbard, like a bokken, is an entirely different roll than falling with a scabbard.

- Constricted falls. Have your partner throw you close enough to a wall or the edge of the mat that you have to adjust your flat fall landing position in the air to land in a safe place.

- Falling counterattack. Counterattack either in the air or immediately on hitting the ground. Twists and drags, especially using hair, are very dangerous—they put a lot of torque on the threat's neck. Practice safely. Most strikes don't have power when you are falling. The most effective counters tend to be sutemi waza, or the judo sacrifice throws.

- Obstacle falls are difficult to set up safely. Once you have falls down well, put a soft obstruction, like a foam brick, in the landing and take a throw. Conform your body in the air to land properly without touching the object.

Pushing

Pushing is not the push-hands drill of some Chinese arts, though I derived this drill from a simple tip from Fabien Sena. You gotta listen to a Belgian guy teaching Chinese martial arts in Tokyo.

There are three elements to hitting hard: power generation, power stealing, and power conservation. Power generation includes all the things you can do with your muscles to make the strike as hard as possible: getting legs behind a punch, adding a hip twitch, and working on arm and hand speed. Power stealing is using either gravity or the threat's momentum to add to the power you are applying to the system.

Power conservation, usually called structure, doesn't add anything to the system. It is plugging the leaks in energy transfer so that as much of the energy as possible is transmitted to the bad guy.

Concept: For our purposes, the body is composed of bones wrapped in meat, or muscle. Muscle without bone is limp. You can slap with it, but if you want to penetrate, you have to hit with bone. A bone is like any other rigid object, like a stick: the straighter it is on the line of force applied, the less likely it is to bend, break, or twist away.

Bones, in addition, are multiple. The straight line along the line of applied force can never be perfectly straight because it is coming from your legs vertically and out your arm horizontally. The next best thing to a straight line is a good architectural arch.

Each connection between two bones in the power chain, each joint, is a potential place to lose power.

Pushing is a simple way to check your structure and see where power is being lost.

Do this: the exercise is simple. At the impact point of any strike, you memorize the position, the feel of exactly where your feet, legs, spine, and arms are, and you then go to a rigid structure like a wall and re-create the position.

You put power into the action, pushing against the wall, and feel.

If you are pushing yourself back, your power arch is broken, with the angles too sharp. If your spine rotates, it probably wasn't rotated enough toward the target at the moment of impact (and learning this can actually give you a couple of inches of range). If your heels are up and the push puts you back down, you were sacrificing a little power for speed. You have to decide if it is worth the trade.

The idea is that the more power you put in your technique, the more solidly you feel forced directly into the ground. No bending, no twisting, no swaying.

You will find out a lot about power as you do this drill with different strikes and at odd angles. Slight twists in forearm alignment can make a noticeable difference. Very close techniques at an upward angle are very strong linearly, whereas long-range hand techniques often have a slight downward vector, creating an arch.

You can maintain power at some very weird angles, with a little practice, like bent over with your spine twisted. It won't be as strong as your good set strikes, but it will be stronger than most people expect or might even believe is possible.

If good body mechanics are used (power generation) and you exploit your weight, the threat's motion (power stealing), or both, there is an enormous amount of force in a decent strike. The only reason most hits are not extremely devastating is because so much power is lost to inefficient structure.

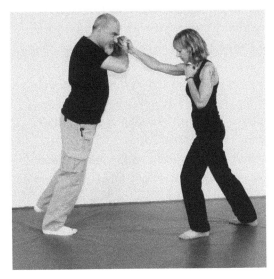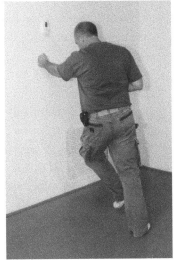

Structure Check

Core Defense

Have fun with this one because in a lot of ways, it is more a game than a drill. It requires a partner.

Do this: the person doing the drill, practicing core defense, crosses his wrists over his chest. He then keeps his hands in that position. If necessary, he grabs his own shirt. The partner then begins throwing punches, slowly at first. This must be done from good punching range. The punches should include the full repertoire of hand strikes: jabs, hooks, chops, ridges, uppercuts, crosses . . . the works.

The defender protects himself with dodging, slipping, and, most important for this drill, shoulder and elbow blocks and glides. Shrugging is one of the great and easy infighting defenses.

The drill has multiple functions. As a physical skill, defending without relying on hand speed is critical in a close-range fight. When the hands are in, the elbows are already in a position to protect the ribs without extraneous movement. Slight shifts with your shoulders are very effective for protecting the head. These are infighting techniques and the ability to use your shoulders, elbows, and hips (yup, they come into play too) defensively while keeping your major offensive weapons free is a huge edge. In infighting, efficiency and (I need a single word here for quick adaptability combined with a broad awareness of both everything that is happening and all the possibilities in the system) are king.

As a mental drill, as the partner speeds up and increases power, you get used to being in the eye of the storm. If you haven't experienced it, it can be overwhelmingly chaotic. With just a taste, it is manageable. With some practice, you own the center of the storm.

There is also a transition built into the drill. As the flurries come in faster, you need to buy time, and you will naturally find yourself hip slamming or shoulder slamming your partner. This teaches a number of things:

- An offensive move, like a slam, can have incredible defensive ability.

- You can be on the offensive without using or in addition to using your primary weapons.

- You will also discover that you get a feel for timing and the opponent's momentum and can frequently "glide" an attack in such a way that the opponent loses his balance.

You may use the slam as the signal to switch roles, but it will reward the more aggressive fighter and give him or her less training time with it. On the other hand, it will encourage passive students to be more aggressive.

GM: GROUND MOVEMENT DRILLS

Many police officers get just eight hours of training each year in defensive tactics (DTs). As new problems come to attention, such as the rise in potential arrestees who have had some minimal training in mixed martial arts or grappling, officers want to know what to do.

They simply do not have the time to develop the same skills in the same way as a training martial artist. Fortunately, real fighting is about much more than just technical skills.

Given the limited time frame, officers have to be taught from the brain down. You teach them the principles, and they practice applying the principles. Most sport grapplers are taught from the body up. The drills, concepts, and principles that follow are instinctive to every good grappler, but few would be able to explain in words what they do.

The ground movement series is just what it says: a collection of drills to improve your ability to move someone else in a ground fight. It is neither sport grappling training nor is it more than a bare introduction to one of the primary skills.

Moving a body is a fundamental skill of all fighting, and it is a skill.

Like the one-step, the first drill is done slowly. It is about learning to see in a new way. The drill must not become competitive, and you, as a coach, *must* watch for anyone trying to use technique. Techniques are memorized, but principles and natural motions are simply understood. Memory is too slow to work in an onslaught.

There are some principles you must understand in order to effectively use the ground movement drills.

Balance can be seen as a matter of strong and weak lines. Humans are bipedal creatures, a relatively unstable base. No matter how someone stands, if you draw a line between his feet, that will be a strong line. It will be hard to push him off balance on that line. If you draw a line perpendicular to the strong line, that will be the weak line, and it will be relatively easy to unbalance in that direction.

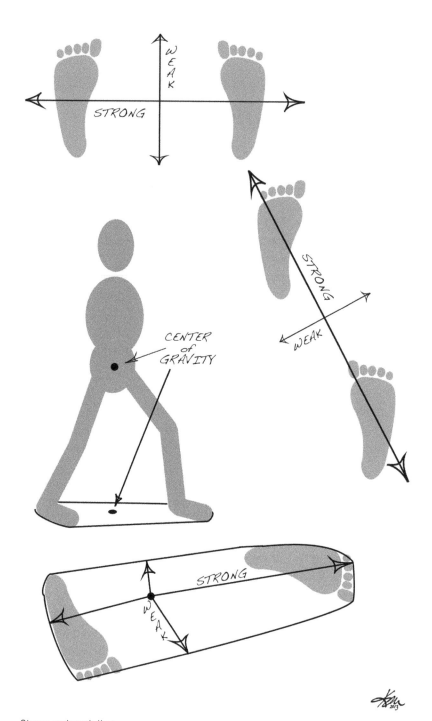

Strong and weak lines

Strong and weak lines are good enough for standing situations, but it is the grade-school version of the real concept.

Your *base* is created by your points of contact with the ground. In the standing example, in most positions, you can draw a line from toe to toe, another line from heel to heel, and use the outside edges of your feet to make a rough rectangle. This is your base. If you are in a "T" stance with the lead toe pointed forward and the rear foot at ninety degrees, your base is a triangle. Conceptually, the base is exactly the same as the base on a chess piece or the little green plastic toy soldiers we played with as kids.

Ground fighting is the reason the strong line/weak line model is inadequate. In a grapple, each point of contact with the ground becomes one of the corners of your base. Connect the dots and you have the shape of the base.

In grappling, a threat in full mount pinning your hands has six points of contact with the ground (both feet, both knees, both hands), making a long rectangle. A threat holding you by the throat and preparing to punch in the mount has five (feet, knees, and the hand on your throat), making a pentagon. A threat in a side headlock or *kesa gatame* position has, at minimum, one shoulder, one hip, the knee and foot of the lower leg, and the foot of the upper leg in contact with the ground and may add more in some variations by putting his head or other hand on the ground.

The center of gravity (CoG) is the point at which your body would balance in all three dimensions. For men it is about a hand's breadth below the navel and between the hip bones. In women it is slightly lower. The CoG has gained some spiritual weight as the *dan tian* and the *hara* or "seat of the hara." Source of *qi* . . . blah, blah, blah.

If the CoG leaves the base provided by your feet, you lose your balance. If you cannot get a foot under it in time to extend your base and keep the CoG inside the bounds, you fall. That simple. That is what losing balance *is*. That is what falling *is*.

And if you can get the threat's CoG outside his base in a grappling situation, he rolls to that side. The principles are simple. Making them happen takes skill.

Rollover

Do this: emphasize that this is a noncompetitive drill and should be done slowly. Student A assumes a position on his back on the mat. Student B then puts student A in any hold or pin (no joint locks or pressure points). Student A then mentally maps student B's points of contact and CoG and decides which direction would be easiest to roll her. That will be whichever edge of the base the CoG is closest to. Moving a body four inches is easier and quicker than moving a body twelve inches.

Once student A finds the easiest direction, student A rolls student B off. Student B does not resist. Then student A takes any hold, and student B rolls him off.

The drill is simple.

Coaching points:

- You will find that some people will try to use specific techniques to escape specific holds or try to use layered strategies to escape. This is game thinking. They need to just learn to see the easy way.

- The person doing the pin is *not* to try to hold on. He or she does not adjust the base or try to wrap so student A is pushing against his own structure.

- You will need to point out that sometimes the easiest direction to roll a threat does not coincide with strong muscle groups, and the student may have to choose a less efficient option that can be applied with more power.

- More leverage can be placed on bone than on squishy places. Unless the leverage or direction is bad, pushing directly on the pelvis is more effective than pushing on the belly.

- Ensure that the student is not in his or her own way, such as having a leg under the direction the person needs to roll, acting as a chock block.

This is not fighting. This is not even wrestling. This is a drill to help the students learn to see the easy way. Just learning to see.

Rollover, Phase 2

There is more to any fight than any single principle. A good grappling contest is a chess match of balance and momentum, altering your opponent's base while changing your own base as necessary, fluidly and dynamically. The last phase is a critical piece, but it is only a piece. Here we add the next one.

Do this: the basics of the drill are the same. In a noncompetitive environment, the person on the bottom tries to find the easiest direction to roll the person on top. In this version, however, you are allowed to change the shape of the base.

I usually demonstrate this from a full mount with wrists pinned. It is a position most women fear and one that allows you to demonstrate two important concepts.

The first concept, not directly related to this drill, is the idea of "fighting emptiness" (see D3: "The Hole against the Wall" for more information). In this position, most people struggle against the force. The wrists are pinned to the ground and the instinct is to attempt to raise them off the ground. That is difficult (impossible with a bigger, stronger threat), but even more, it is useless. However, the arms pinning the wrists can be easily moved merely by sliding the arms along the ground.

Sliding both down quickly causes the threat to lose his balance and fall forward, directly into a headbutt, if the person on the bottom wishes.

That is the key to the concept at the center of this version of the drill. By sliding the arms down, the threat's base changes, and he loses his balance.

The essence of this version is the same as D1, except for the opportunity to change the base. If you can knock a bracing arm away or push a knee straight, the direction to roll will not only change but likely become easier.

Coaching points:

- For some reason, sometimes people will move counter to their own actions, like opening up a hole on the left and moving to the right. That will, obviously, fail.

- Do not forget the basic (GM1) drill. If you can't alter the base, there is still a weak line.

- Just because you move something does not make it better. In the wrist pin example, if the person on the bottom just brings the hands out to the sides, she has actually made a wider and stabler base. The base manipulation must serve the purpose or it is useless.

- Like any principle, there are limits. A lever may allow you to triple your power, but someone who can move only twenty pounds will be able to move only sixty pounds with that lever. Same here. The technique makes things easier; it does not magically make things work. Understand the difference.

- Because of that, GM1 and GM2 may not require partners of roughly equal size, but it will be easier and less frustrating if weight classes are respected. Not that "easy and less frustrating" is always a legitimate goal.

Rollover, Phase 3

The essences of balance are the base and the CoG. The first drill explored those statically. The second drill worked with altering the base. Logically, the next phase will involve manipulating the CoG.

This is another one I demonstrate to illustrate two principles, one general and one specific to the drill.

Do this: we start from the "ground and pound." The threat straddles the student to throw punches at the unprotected face. I have been told by one of the best grapplers in the world that this is the "worst-case scenario." If it makes your top ten, you need to get out more. In training and sport, it is a very bad place to be. Surprisingly, in real life if you keep your head, it's not bad at all.

This goes back to the concept of "gifts" explained in the environmental fighting drill (OS7). If a real bad guy has you down in the ground and pound, how will he hit? With power and speed and murderous intent, most likely. Good. And where will this happen? I can't guarantee asphalt or concrete, but I can pretty much guarantee it won't happen on a nice soft mat.

When that power punch comes at your head, you just need to make him miss by an inch or two. A slight shift of your hips will do it, even if you are far outmatched in size and strength. When his power strike hits the asphalt next to your head, that is one hand he won't use again without surgery.

It's not hard, and the lesson is this: many scary situations are tools if you use them. See. Exploit.

For the purpose of the drill, the principle is a little deeper and correlates with the hole on the wall drill (D3), dynamic fighting (D1), and blindfolded defense (B1). You cannot move without shifting your CoG. The bad guy cannot move—he cannot punch or shift or transition to a hold or submission without moving his CoG. When he does it, he will move it closer to one edge of his base, and he will do it more easily than you could force it. Your enemy's movement is a gift to you.

Because what follows is very dynamic, it is hard for the students not to get competitive. Remind them. This is also a drill where size matters far less.

You can start the drill from the ground and pound if you wish. As the person on top strikes, the other uses the force to unbalance and roll and then moves to a hold or pin position. *Before* he gets in position, the first student uses the motion to keep the roll going and gets on top. Before the first student consolidates, the second keeps the roll going and so on.

Coaching points:

- Because this is dynamic, people with grappling training will try to revert to memorized techniques. Prevent it. The principles are in the drill and usually purer. If they stick with the drill and develop sensitivity to base, CoG, and momentum, their technique will improve.

- You will need one designated safety person, and a lot of room, for each pair.

- Let them hit walls and encourage them to utilize the bounce.

- If anyone gets stuck (loses momentum), just revert to the last two phases: find the easy line or change the base.

- In this drill you can fake. The person will subconsciously try to recover balance, and if the person on the bottom is sensitive, you can ride the recovery and roll the other direction.

Once this drill starts going, you will notice immediately that it looks a lot more like a bar brawl than a grappling contest. That's good. The students need to get used to the dynamics of rapid, nonsport rolling. Even highly skilled people tend to default to brawling (rolling on the floor, throwing wild punches) in a real fight. So it seems it makes sense to practice rolling around on the floor and getting wild. If you are going to go caveman anyway, you might as well be skilled at it.

It also becomes quickly apparent that size and strength are much less important in a dynamic situation than in a static one. The bigger, stronger person supplies the drive, but the smarter person ends up steering. That is power if you use the gift.

Rollover, Phase 4   GM4

This is preceded by a class, and the students have no idea that we are going to return to the ground. The class is on pain. I explain the ethics, use, and limitations of pain. Then explain, if it is unfamiliar to them, the concept of stacking.

Stacking is using multiple techniques or types of techniques simultaneously. For instance, (techniques) a shoulder lock with a finger lock so that the person can't move in either direction or (types of techniques) using a pressure point to set up a sweep and then a kick to execute it (movement, pain, and damage all combined in a single technique).

We then proceed to a few of the more practical pain points. For this purpose, practical points are those that normally cause a reliable and useful reaction.

The ones I typically show are as follows:

- Mandibular
- Submandibular
- Supraphiltrum
- Jaw hinge
- Suprasternal notch
- Pectoral
- Lats
- Axillary
- Intercostals
- Golgi reflex tendon
- Radial
- Inguinal
- Inner thigh
- Tip of the fibula
- Achilles lock

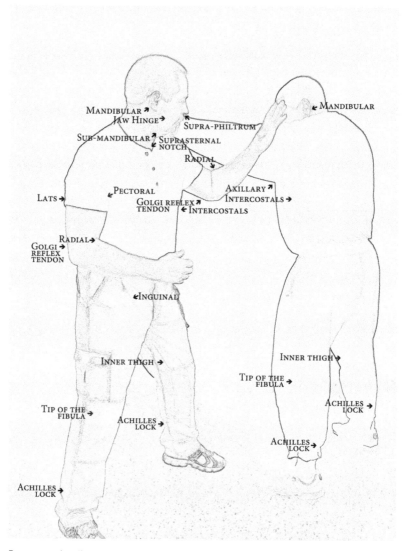

Pressure point diagram

Do this: after this class, when everyone has found the relevant points, we begin the phase-4 drill. The drill is exactly the same as the phase 3, but the person on the bottom is allowed to use pressure points to further unbalance the one on top.

It makes things much easier.

A note: It is not a drill, but after this progression, I usually teach a short class on striking from the ground. The class must cover how to generate power, appropriate weapons, and targets. Striking well from the ground is one of the primary tools in a brawl and blends well with the skills already developed in moving a body.

The Wax On, Wax Off of Ground Fighting   GM

There are two moves that are the "wax on, wax off" of ground fighting.

Do this: the first is the hip arch. When you are lying on your back, you bring your feet as close to your butt as possible and explosively launch your hips as high as you can. It is a strong muscle group and can often launch a bigger person off of you.

It should be practiced frequently, and the relevant muscles can be trained with back and neck bridges.

Slightly changing the power coming from each leg and working your hips allow you to launch the threat at an angle. You can even aim him.

Then do this: the second is the shrimp or *ebi*. Lying on your side, you bring your elbow and knee together, which drags your lower body up. You extend your body as you roll to the other side and again bring your knee to your elbow.

The shrimp is a good defensive position that coils your core for explosive motion. As you do the drill, you will make distance across the training floor. It should be practiced regularly, and you can do shrimp races.

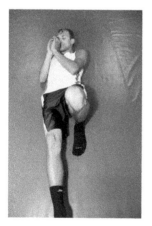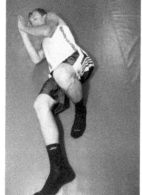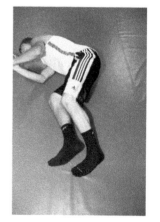

Ebi or shrimping

One Up, One Down GM6

This is not an exercise to move another person so much as to familiarize with how to move on the ground when it is unsafe to stand.

Do this: one person will be standing, the other down. The person in the down position will be in roughly the formal position for a side flat fall (*yoko ukemi*) with the down leg bent, rolled onto one side, the other leg raised and coiled, the down arm on the ground, and the other arm raised to defend the face (which is probably unnecessary).

The standing partner will attempt to close with the down partner.

Because the upper leg is not based and has no weight on it, it doesn't present a good target. As long as the down person's legs stay between her and the threat, she has no good targets below the crotch. That means the standing threat cannot close against the legs without exposing his knees or his own crotch to a devastating stamping kick.

From the down position, the key to the drill is to keep your legs between you and the threat. The threat will try to circle, fake, and close. You will keep him at bay with taps on his knee whenever he is in range. From the down position, you must practice circling and, if he fakes you good, flipping from right to left sides to cover large distances (almost ninety degrees).

When it is time to switch, the person down uses the opportunity to practice standing safely—keeping the eyes on the threat, rolling forward so the top leg comes to the ground, hand up to protect the face, ready to roll back into the ground defense position immediately if the threat reengages. Then smoothly pressing up to stand when the feet are both under the CoG and the base is stable.

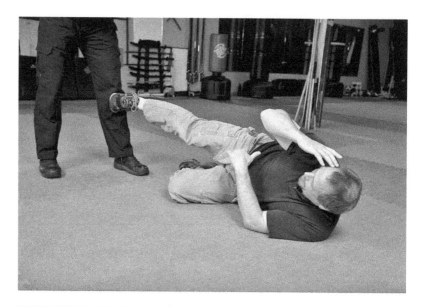

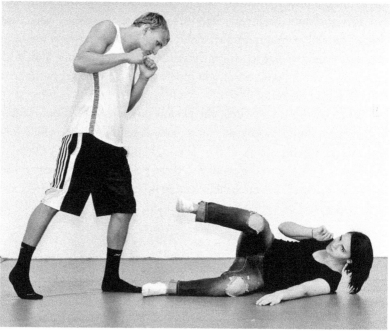

One up, one down position

Blindfolded Grappling
GM7

Do this: if grappling is part of your regular training, practice blind-folded. You will need safety monitors, especially if you have active rollers, to keep them from rolling into other groups or hard objects. If there are no corners, I like my guys to get the opportunity to roll into walls and use them.

This is grappling, not ground fighting. Using strikes or weapons raises the level of risk significantly. Movement, immobilizations, locks (except spine), pressure points, and strangles are all easy to do and relatively safe to practice blindfolded. Many practitioners find that blindfolded work is easier and smoother than seeing.

For the record, you can do two-on-one blindfolded grappling with just you blindfolded. (Your two opponents need to see so they can work together and they don't start accidentally fighting each other.) It is exhausting, but educational and fun.

INTERLUDE #3:
SOCIAL AND ASOCIAL

I'm not going to recap the breakdowns. Social and asocial violence and the subgroups are pretty thoroughly described in *Facing Violence*.

Quick recap: Social violence is what we do to people; asocial is what we do to animals.

If you are going to kill an animal, do you need to get worked up, to get angry? Do you need to convince yourself this cow is a bad cow and deserves to die? You have a reason to kill (food)—do you also need a justification, like justice? Does it occur to you to give the cow a chance? Do you fight the cow or simply kill it?

When humans apply asocial violence, it is quick and clean and easy. Maybe a little emotional the first couple of times. But a man with a knife can safely and in a matter of seconds kill a two-hundred-pound hog.

Turn the same man with a knife on a person and it tends to get all kinds of messy.

Generally, people need to be worked up and angry to do harm to another person. Angry people make mistakes. Reasons aren't enough. Very, very few people can say, "I needed to stop him from hurting me" and just stop there. They need to add how bad the person was or why it was morally right. It clogs the brain with bullshit at a time when you really can't afford it. And almost always, in self-defense, people fight other people instead of just taking them out.

Experienced violent criminals have gotten past this and can treat people like animals, which gives them a huge advantage. The person defending herself usually cannot.

This has other implications. If you are in social "fight" mode, you will subconsciously be hitting to communicate, not to eliminate. You might have every intention of an open-handed shot to the brainstem or ear and find yourself turning it into a punch to the jaw at the last second. You probably know well that a powerful strike is loose and smooth, but you will tense up and pull at the last minute because you are subconsciously trying to send a dominance message, and you dominate better if you are tensed up, looking big.

These are subconscious tendencies that can torpedo you if you are ever attacked, but there are more. Many martial styles developed from dueling systems in which dominance is the point. Square off, prove who is the better man . . .

And so these systems work very well in monkey dances, which you can always walk away from. And people almost never get injured in monkey dances. Superb skills for situations with no risk that you can avoid anyway.

It is easier to take someone out from behind. So obvious I am embarrassed to write it. So how often do you practice getting behind? Do you have tools to finish from there, like cervical spine strikes?

Most important, and what I am trying to say: do you honestly train to take people out? To go into an asocial mode and just finish this? Or do you train for a social fight?

This is critical. Even worse than the fact that most social violence does minimal injury, social violence is almost completely scripted. If you are trying to defend yourself with your brain in social mode, you will not injure the threat and you are 100 percent predictable.

And bad guys know this. They will do everything in their power to keep a victim in social mode, from talking to arguing to bargaining. They know that if you are scared badly enough, you will fight like a panicked animal. If you can go completely cold, you might be smarter than the bad guy. But if you are in communicating mode, you are a completely predictable and completely safe victim.

You must train for going asocial. That doesn't mean ultraviolent, but it does become ultra-efficient. Putting handcuffs on is just getting a job done. Not a fight, not a contest.

PM: THE PLASTIC-MIND
EXERCISES

Martial arts are often taught as movement exercises. In a very real sense a good martial artist has trained in a stylized way to play with his or her body. Just like a dancer, gymnast, or free runner. Movement is a critical skill for enjoying life. Movement is fun. Your own body is the second-best toy you will ever have.

The best toy is your mind.

Personality, identity, ego—the sense of who we are—is not as solid as we like to think. Are you the same person after forty hours without sleep? Decreasing animal protein in your diet messes with serotonin levels. I'm not even the same person before my second cup of coffee.

One of the greatest delusions in self-defense training is the unstated belief that if you ever have to use your skills, you will, somehow, undergo the most intense fifteen seconds of your life without changing.

You will change. Profoundly. Change is not bad. Fear of change usually is.

The plastic-mind exercises are ways to play with your mind and personality in a martial context. Will they turn you into a different person? Maybe, maybe not, but they will show you the possibility is there and you can take conscious control. For a few critical moments in your life you can choose who you need to be.

Most of the plastic-mind drills will play from the one-step drill to allow for time to think and to ensure safety.

PM1 and 2 get to the essence of what a martial system truly is. All martial systems, all styles, are merely integrated systems of movement. The more cleanly the system is integrated, the more efficiently it will work and the faster it will be to learn.

Integration means it works together. Techniques must serve tactics and tactics must serve strategies and strategies must serve your goals. If any of those is unknown or undefined, everything loses focus.

If you are a peaceful person and therefore your primary strategy in self-defense is to escape . . . but since you are peaceful and don't

want to injure anyone, your primary tactics center on joint locks ...
it's a problem. Because you can't simultaneously lock someone's joints
and leave.

If your goal is clear, and your strategy is clear and serves your
goals, it often makes your tactics obvious.

"To integrate ourselves and the enemy with the infinite power of
the universe to achieve a harmonious outcome with minimal harm"
might sound cool and maybe logical, and it even has the word *integrate*
in it. But it is fuzzy and unwieldy and thus profoundly unintegrated.

"Him down now." That's integrated and tells you most of what
you need to know.

Animal Styles

Animal styles are big in the Chinese systems. It's abundantly clear that the monks who created the systems were shitty observers: the crane movements look much more like the wing and leg movements of a mating dance than the sneaking and short jabbing bites into a fish's back that a crane actually uses . . . but the concept is important.

This isn't about reality. This is about the way the mind works. The animals in the mind are myths, representations, not biologically accurate entities. They are ideas that influence your thought and movement.

Do this: to conduct the drill, have each student choose and imagine an animal. There are potential advantages to naming the animal out loud in that it can reinforce the concept, but usually they keep it to themselves.

Then, fighting as two different animals, the students begin the one-step.

Coaching tips:

- After a round of a few minutes, ask the student's to identify the opponent's animal.

- Let them tell you how much their basic movement patterns changed.

- Ask, "Who found themselves thinking differently?" and listen.

- If people go for the regular martial animals—monkey, bear, crane, snake—suggest some off-the-wall ones: ram, squirrel, mouse, octopus, orca. The point is to push the limits of your own mind, not re-create someone else's ideas.

After the first round, have them trade partners and either try a new animal or stay with the same one, but if they stay with the same partner, they change animals.

Fighting the Elements   PM

Do this: in this variation, each student will make up four entirely new and entirely coherent martial arts. Have them imagine the four alchemical elements of earth, wind, fire, and water.

At the next round of one-step, each student is to choose one of the elements, his partner chooses another, and they begin the drill. Each will fight the way she imagines a master of the earth or fire or wind or water style would fight. Real earth would just lie there, and fire would run uphill and downwind . . . but they resonate as symbols, and in the symbols are keys to thinking and movement, even strategy and technique.

Tell the students that they will be fighting as masters of one of these ancient, elemental styles.

As you observe, you will see every last student working with what is clearly a unique martial system that was entirely invented in under a minute.

The brain is a powerful integrator with the right concept.

Have the partners stay together and choose a new element for the next round. Repeat until each person has represented all four elements. Then let them debrief and talk about what they did, thought, and especially felt. What did wind feel like? How well did it work? Did one element feel more natural than the others?

Did they feel like they were creating a system or stepping into one that was ready-made? Did it feel like inventing, remembering, or something else?

It is critically important in debriefing any of the plastic-mind exercises for the instructor *not* to be directive. This is a gentle exploration of the student's mind, conducted by the student. If the instructor tells a student what he felt or what she experienced, right or wrong it will become an assumption and a preconception. Let the students explore and play.

And for you, instructor: there is a fifth element, sometimes called "the void." How would you fight as the void?

The Other   PM3

Throughout the one-step, throughout all of your training, there has been a subconscious assumption. The assumption has been slightly different for different students. In almost every instance where people were going too fast, cheating on the drill, and not maintaining control, one or both partners were thinking of the other as an opponent. When the drill was going well, they were thinking of each other as training partners. It is time to bring those thoughts to the surface and play with them.

Do this: the most senior, experienced, or skillful partner in each pair is instructed to change nothing. Just continue to do the one-step as always.

The junior member begins the first round with this instruction: "You have been doing the one-step with your training partner all day. Now I want you to do it with your enemy. Stay slow, stay controlled, but this is the person who killed your child or your parents. Begin."

This may require extra safety monitors. Watch the change in intensity, the change in choice of techniques. In debriefing, have the students explain what they felt and noticed. How they moved differently.

The next round: "You are the teacher, and you are sparring (one-step) with a not-very-bright student. Without using words, show them what the drill should be. Begin."

Same debriefing. Notice how the quality of the entire interaction is noticeably different. During debriefing, have the seniors, who theoretically didn't change, describe what it is like to be on the receiving end of the different personalities.

Next, "You are a big playful cat. The other person isn't a person at all. He is a big cat toy. Your cat toy. Play." This gets some of the most interesting changes. People of a relatively low skill level often start casually dominating a far more skilled martial artist.

"Your opponent is your servant. Everything he does is a gift for you. If he hits your jaw, it just puts more power in your own strike as you spin with it. He is a part of your machine, and you own it all."

"Fight him like Mother Teresa. You are there to help him."

"Fight like you are invulnerable."

Each of these experiments (and as many more as you can imagine, just don't burn out the students) causes deep changes in strategy, tactics, and techniques. People fight differently when they think about themselves or the opponent in different ways. This can be exploited.

It is too much to go into in a short book of drills, but buried in this drill are the concepts to becoming a supremely ethical fighter (or the opposite), a singularly controlled or wild fighter, focused or calm.

Up until the age of six or so, we all played versions of this game and pretended to be knights or wild animals or cowboys, and for those moments, with a child's purity of intent, we were those things. We could be as tough as John Wayne or as self-sacrificing as Galahad ... as long as no one reminded us we were just children. The powers of imagination—and the greater powers of pure intent and belief—are still there. Most of us have just gotten a little rusty.

IW: INTERNAL WORK

Fighting is an aspect of living. If you live poorly—weak and slow and unobservant—you will fight poorly. Fighting arises from your nature.

Nature is not immutable. You grow all the time. You have already experienced vast changes in your life (puberty, anyone?), and you will certainly experience more. Even more than that, many aspects of your identity will change depending on sleep deprivation, dehydration, or low blood sugar.

Your base personality will change even more under fear, pain, and stress. To know you are a different person before and after your second cup of coffee but to believe that you will go through an assault unchanged is not only arrogant but childish.

People change and grow over time, especially curious people and active people. But, except in extreme conditions, it rarely happens quickly . . . and don't get your hopes up about the extreme conditions. When the stress is on, you will do worse, not better, than you are used to. Finding a hero buried somewhere in your psyche is a myth.

You change by building habits and by spending time around people you admire. You will raise (or lower) your game to fit with the people you hang out with, so pick the best. For that matter, look around right now. If all of your friends are losers, so are you.

The drills that follow work on your senses, your internal self, and your interactions with the world.

Centering

I picked this up from *Psychological First Aid: Field Operations Guide*. It was recommended as a way to calm down children who had lost everything in natural or man-made disasters.

It also turns out to be really good meditation, a way to get in touch with the world, and a way to hone your senses.

Do this: when you practice this, first shut your eyes.

Next name five things you hear:

Traffic on a distant highway.
A truck starting in the other direction.
Wind rattling the aspen leaves.
Birds in three directions.
A strange, hard-to-hear whine from above and behind. Maybe an exhaust fan on the building roof?

Name five things you feel:

The breeze over my ears.
Hard wood of the picnic table bench under my ass.
A bandage tugging at my lower back.
My teeth against my tongue.
Shirt resting on my shoulders.

Name five things you smell:

This is the hardest and not in the original exercise. We don't have good vocabularies for smells, and that makes them hard to register consciously. Smells are subtle as well. You'll have to work at it.

Something that smells like bubblegum.
Wet soil, but faint.
My own teeth. Ick.
Car exhaust, but faint as well.

Something that smells "green." Probably the bushes right behind (upwind) from me.

Yeah. I broke off a leaf to check. That's the smell.

The centering drill is calming. It was originally a technique for extreme stress. It forces you into your senses, into your physical body. It makes you engage with the world. *What is that humming noise? What is the smell beneath the smell?*

Eating Frogs

One of the most catastrophic failures in self-defense is to do nothing. There are many ways to freeze, many reasons people take damage or acquiesce to attackers. Sometimes they feel they need a plan. Sometimes they are in denial that the event is happening. Rarely the victim doesn't know what to do. Often the victim does know what to do but can't seem to make himself or herself do it.

Fighting is unpleasant. It hurts, for one thing. You have to get very close, touching close, to people you would normally avoid. It can smell bad, and there is the definite possibility of messy spills.

You won't enjoy defending yourself from an assault.

Do this: make it a habit to do the things you don't enjoy. Immediately, efficiently, and without hesitation.

If you are going to jump in the cold water, jump. Don't work yourself up to it. As long as it is safe (the water is deep enough, no rocks . . .), jump. Jump with your whole heart.

If you study martial arts and think there is an aspect of training that is useless or that you hate, do it. Do it until those feelings go away. If you think that kata is useless and boring, excellent. Facing that boredom is the center of self-discipline.

If the very idea of competing in a tournament makes you nervous, you must do it. That is fear, a low-level fear, and facing fear is the essence of self-defense.

Everyone should experience rough impact. Microconcussions are bad, and I don't recommend people box for long, but everyone who is interested not just in self-defense but also in who he or she really is should experience boxing. Taking a hit, keeping cool or finding useful emotional triggers (either can work, and both have limitations), and staying in the fight are invaluable skills.

So what is this drill, frog eating? It is a habit. From this moment forward if there is something that needs to be done, you do it. Decisively and immediately.

Constantly feel for your own glitches—the things you fear or hate or that disgust you. If something is unpleasant, at any level, do that first. Kill it. Without hesitation.

I honestly don't know how much this habit crosses over to self-defense. There is a lot of training that doesn't help in a first encounter (where the unfamiliarity can be overwhelming—you don't even know what you are seeing) that really helps in future encounters. This might be one of the ones that helped me, even the first time, because I remember so vividly forcing myself to go hands-on.

But like most of the life skills presented here, there is no downside. What will your boss think of someone who does the hard stuff first and without complaining? Will your family appreciate a you who gets stuff done? Will you be setting an example to be proud of?

And personally, humans are afraid of what they do not know. Because of the fear, they keep away from the situations where they could learn. It makes for a spiral of ignorance and fear feeding each other. As you do things you are afraid of, maybe even your own taxes, you will learn and see how little there is in the world that is actually dangerous.

Not only does this drill make you tougher, but it also makes you smarter and, in the end, wiser. The person who acts when everyone else hesitates is a hero. Eating frogs becomes a superpower.

The Game of the Stones

This came originally from Rudyard Kipling's book *Kim*. The essence is simple.

Do this: get a box. Have someone put various items in the box. You look at those items for a short time, close the box, and then name all the items and where they were in the box.

There are two variables in the simple game: the number of items and how long you look. Human short-term memory usually handles five to nine things. That's OK for seven-digit phone numbers. Most of us can remember one for long enough to dial or quickly get a license plate for long enough to write it down.

Start with seven items. When that becomes easy, add two. Then two more. Then don't add any but put in eleven entirely new items and see if it is still easy. You can keep going as far as you can take it.

You can also decrease the time, and the ideal is to get as much information as possible with a glance.

There are variations in drills for the Real World™. The game of the stones allows for an almost infinite variety. Right now, describe your neighbor's house in detail: color, roof shape, number of windows on each wall, number and location of chimneys and vents, roof composition. If you have been inside, draw a map. Draw a map of the yard.

This habit of scanning places will help immeasurably if you ever have to escape from an area. Where are the exits? Where are the fire extinguishers? Can the walls, windows, or doors be smashed through if necessary? Where are the breaker switches and the gas and water shutoffs? You should know this about the places you spend much time, but you will have to get a feel for it in places you are only passing through.

Same with people. What is every member of your family wearing right now? If one of them disappeared, that is critical information. "Blondish-brown hair and really cute" is hard to search for in a crowd. A yellow hoodie is easier.

Next time you are in a restaurant, on a bus, or in any crowded place, play the game of the stones, using the people around you as stones. After you take your seat, from memory, describe all the people, what they were wearing, and where they were located.

You will not be good at this right away. It's actually sort of appalling how unobservant we all are. That's OK. Like most drills and exercises, there is a practice effect. The more you do something, the better you get at it.

Lists

IV

The bucket list is a list of things you want to do before you kick the bucket. I first heard of it as "fifty things to do before I die."

I'm not sure the specific number is important. Before you read to the end of this section, make a list. Fifty is a good number. You have a great life if you can think of only twenty things you want to do. This is the list of things to do. We'll talk about it later. Make the list before you read further, unless you are into cheating and want to negate the effects of this drill.

Do this: now make a list of your fears. Not the rational fears—I'm afraid of getting shot and I have no intention of shooting myself to get over it. If your fear is a fear because it would be stupid not to be afraid, you can leave it off the list. For this list I want the things that make your hands sweaty and you aren't sure why: singing or speaking in public, dank basements, heights, flames, murky water.

When I was four or five years old, we had a cabin on the Little Deschutes River in Oregon. It had forests, a swimming hole, and even a swamp. I overheard my parents saying one of the other property owners was thinking about getting rid of his kid's pet baby alligator (you could buy them in pet shops at the time) by letting it go in the swamp.

I had nightmares and started to avoid the river.

For years, the one irrational fear I was aware of was murky water. The adrenaline in body surfing never came from the rush of waves and the crash; it was always because of the potential for things with teeth, invisible in the water.

Over twenty years later, my National Guard unit was in Ecuador, providing medical services to villages. We needed to swim a container of dental equipment across a tributary of the Rio Napo, which was itself a tributary of the Amazon. Murky water in the land of all my childhood fears: piranhas, caimans, and anacondas . . .

I volunteered. It was the scariest thing I had ever done. So I needed to do it.

Make the list of fears. There will be patterns. The common pattern is that people are more afraid of embarrassment than of injury or even death. Part of this drill is not to go out and face your fears (though that is perfectly fine as well, and great training) but to learn a little about yourself. About your patterns.

There is a profound difference between fear management and danger management.

Danger or risk management is about not getting hurt. It requires an objective assessment of the situation, as much intelligence as you can gather in whatever time you have, and training and equipment that are relevant to the situation.[2]

Fear management is about feelings, and these feelings are largely imaginary. A black belt can make you feel safer, but in the end, it is a strip of cloth. A rabbit's foot can also make you feel safer.

Good training can make you safer; any training, good or bad, can make you feel safer.

So read your list of fears and look for patterns. Then start pushing at the fears that are imaginary or social. Distinguish between the fear and danger on the list, and challenge the fears.

This is critical. Most conflict we have been exposed to in our culture is social. We have seen dominance games in locker rooms and around the dinner table. We have cold-shouldered the outsider who tried to break into our clique or been the ostracized outsider. Many of us were spanked as children or "thwapped" on the back of the head when we transgressed the rules of the group.

We are used to this social level of conflict. It has rules we have absorbed since our first breath. When it escalates to physical violence, it also follows certain rules, and we count on those:

- There is a clear escalation.

- There are ways to de-escalate from the violence, like apologizing.

---

[2] That right there differentiates good self-defense from bad self-defense training. Accurate assessment ("How do attacks happen?") and training specifically for the realistic problem.

- In most situations, there is a limit to the amount of physical damage that will be done. We have all been taught that if we cry "uncle," the violence will stop.

Predators, experienced violent criminals, and those who have taken violence as part of their identity do *not* follow these rules. But they expect their victims to follow them, and often the victims do.

A predator can transition to violence with no visible escalation . . . and the victim freezes, thinking, "Where did that come from?"

The social de-escalation strategies will backfire with a predator. As long as you are dealing with things socially, the predator knows you are completely predictable and you will not use extreme force, one of the few things he fears.

And the predator will stop when he gets what he wants, not when you acknowledge his dominance.

Breaking your own social rules is a huge element of successful self-defense. If public speaking is hard, how much harder will hitting a stranger be? You have absorbed both of those taboos since infancy, but I'm willing to bet that you have spoken in public at least a couple of times before.

That is the value of the fear list. Breaking your social conditioning as an act of will. The same things that turn you into a babbling idiot when you ask someone on a date or make your voice seem whining when you argue that you deserve a raise are the same category of fear and social programming that will make you hit with half force the first time you are attacked.

The third list is a list of the things you love, but it's not like that. There is often a big gap between who you are and who you think you are. Sometimes the gap is obvious to outsiders.

For the first stage, make a list of the things you love to do and the people you love to spend time with.

For the second stage, you'll need to keep a notebook with you for at least a week. For a minimum of one week, keep track of how you actually spend your time. How many hours you spend at each place, doing each thing with each person.

Compare the lists. The list of things you love? That is who you think you are or, at best, wish to be. The second list is who you are. Sucks? Get over it.

If you say you love your family and spend zero time with them, that's a pretty damn weird definition of love. If you spend more time drinking with the guys from work and complaining about the job, that complaining is more important to you, more important to your identity, than your family.

I'll cut you some slack for sleeping and for working—you need to pay for other things you love. But otherwise, no matter how painful, the second list is a solid indicator of who you really are.

If there is a big gap between the lists, you have four options. First, you can shrug and say, "So what?" and continue living with a big separation between belief and action. It's way too common.

Or you can change your life to bring it closer to your vision. Start doing what you say you love.

Or you can learn to love what you are doing, bring your vision closer to your life.

Or you can do both of the last two.

Now, back to the first list, the list of things you want to do. Yeah, yeah, do as many as you can in the time you have, blah, blah, blah. That's pretty much a platitude. Here is the value of that list:

Which of those things could you have already done? And why didn't you? Almost everything on that list is possible. Were you willing to make sacrifices? A five-dollar latte once a day adds up to $1,825 a year. Two, maybe three years of that is a cruise, a diving trip to Central America . . . less than a year for skydiving lessons.

Why didn't you? This is important because almost nothing you say will be a reason. Almost all will be excuses. If you want to know the difference, ask a smart person to brainstorm with you how to accomplish a few things on your list. When you say, "I can't because . . ." and they shoot it down or find a work-around, you were offering an excuse.

The value in this drill is to find your habitual excuses to avoid improving your life. *It's too expensive.* Look at your junk food bill or, for that matter, your cable bill: has anyone ever put "Watch more television" on a bucket list? *I don't have the time.* Look at the amount of time you waste in a day. *I don't know how.* That's what books and classes and the internet are for. Find out how.

This is the final list, the list of your habitual excuses. This is the one that needs to go up on the bathroom mirror as a constant reminder. Whenever you hear these excuses come out of your mouth, it's time to hit the problem or take the opportunity head-on. Decisively. With everything you've got.

Slaughtering and Butchering

Yes. Literally.

If someone trains for a decade or three and his techniques fail, I understand if he is upset. Often, though, when the technique works, the practitioner is equally upset because he was unprepared for the sound of breaking bones and the vision of a big man trying weakly to scream.

One of the biggest disconnects in martial arts training is that it is so easy to forget what you are training to do. An elegant throw is slamming a man's head into the ground with sufficient force to shatter his shoulder or his neck. A powerful, focused punch is concussing the brain and breaking or dislocating the jaw.

This is not mindfulness. To practice and to either forget or ignore what you are practicing is something close to unforgivable.

Hunting is not an adequate illustration of what you need to feel. With bow or rifle, the distance is too great. The connection is missing. The skill going into the stalk becomes the focus—not the death, not the act of killing.

Slaughtering, killing a domestic animal, is a different thing. It is more intense if you have raised the animal, named it, and it is a species you like. I never really liked sheep and slaughtering them doesn't bother me much. I do like goats. They are smart and wild and have personalities. I learn more, and it hits me harder to kill a goat.

Understand this: the point of this exercise is to hit yourself as hard as you legally and ethically can.

Do this: legally kill an animal, not a human; a food animal, not a pet; and one that belongs to you or you have permission to slaughter.

Ethically, you would learn more killing with your bare hands or making a botch of it with a knife, but any unnecessary pain is wrong. When you kill, under any circumstances, it should be as quick, clean, and painless as you can make it. That is the right thing to do.

Most of you reading this will never do this exercise. (Hell, you probably won't do most of them. Just read and think and say, "That's close enough.")

Those who do, your options are to raise your own animal or help out a friend who already butchers. It's nice to have small farmers for friends. It also helps because you will have someone with a proven method to teach you.

I have slaughtered with a gun and a sword.

We had to put down Gazelle, a paralyzed goat. Put down means "kill." Maybe it means "kill for its own good, for the cessation of pain." I went out early in the morning and dug the grave. It is a sin in my family to waste meat, but since the paralysis was probably due to loss of circulation, the meat may not have been safe. I dug the grave close because I know limp bodies are much harder to move than stiff ones. I took aim from about a foot and a half away with a .40 caliber semiautomatic handgun and pulled the trigger.

The shot was very loud in the morning quiet. I'd aimed for the sniper spot, the brainstem. We are taught that in a hostage situation, a direct hit on the brainstem will make the threat go limp, so he will not reflexively clench his hands and pull a trigger. I missed. Live targets move, or I may have rushed the shot out of fear that Gazelle would move. I'm a pretty decent shot with a handgun. That means on my best days I'm about half as good as a TV hero. The round entered about an inch from my aim point, missing the brainstem but entering the brain cavity. It was a special expanding bullet and didn't exit the skull. Gazelle started shuddering and twitching.

She was dead. CSF (cerebral spinal fluid) and blood had erupted from both ears and her nose at the shot. Her eyes were fixed. I touched her eyeball and there was no blink reflex. She was dead, dead, dead. But the brainstem is old and animal and it kept her legs jerking and her heart beating and her breath going in little raspy gasps. For about a minute. I think I watched that long because I was convincing myself she was dead and I didn't screw up. But Kami, my wife, was there (my excuse?), and it was hard on her to watch. (Oh, no, couldn't be hard on me . . . I've been butchering animals since I was a kid! Bullshit. It's still hard. I just do it more efficiently and with more respect and with clearer reasons now.) So I fired again, this time hitting the sniper spot, and Gazelle went limp.

People don't die much differently.

That is the point, of course, and the importance of this exercise. Martial arts and self-defense, on one level, deal in the destruction of the human body. Pretty that up if you have to, but if you need prettier words, you haven't come to terms with what you may need to do.

I could tell you what you might learn about life, about weapons, and about yourself, but I won't. You need to do the drill, produce your own meat, to find out some things.

Ethics and Glitches

IW

Do this: a thought experiment, something you can do just sitting here, reading and thinking. Here is a scenario:

Someone is approaching you with a butcher knife, intent on killing you. You are backed into a corner and have nowhere to retreat. You have a gun. This is a pure shoot/no-shoot scenario. Do you shoot? Or let yourself be killed?

Are you OK with your decision?

Think about that for a second.

What follows are slight changes to the scenario. The questions are always the same. Do you shoot? Are you OK with the decision?

Get this: I don't want answers. Neither do you. As the scenario changes, I want you to notice when you shift feelings—when the decision to shoot is preceded by a slight hesitation, or when you really don't want to think about it.

These hesitations are what I call glitches, the things that might make you freeze in a survival situation. They indicate that you have moral and ethical issues with using force. Congratulations. We all do. But it's a damn good idea to know what they are before someone tries to kill you.

When you find your glitches, don't try to fix them or judge them. Not yet. Just bring them out into the light and examine them.

So, same basic scenario: someone coming at you with a lethal weapon, a fourteen-inch butcher knife. The threat wants to kill you, and you are cornered but armed. Do you shoot? Do you feel OK with it? What if . . .

- the threat is fourteen years old? Twelve? Ten? Six?
- the threat is a woman?
- a pregnant woman?
- your children are watching?
- the threat's children are watching?
- it is someone you love, like a veteran father having a flashback, or your own child suffering from an acute psychotic episode?

- you are being filmed by a news crew?
- the threat is severely developmentally disabled, incapable of knowing what he or she is doing?

Anything you glitched on means something.

This drill just scratches the surface of all the possible glitches and in a way is the mental companion to slaughtering.

To Save My Children IW

Do this: yet another thought experiment and one incredibly relevant to modern self-defense:

If no one were going to help you and there were a very real possibility your children would starve tomorrow, what would you be willing to do?

Would you steal? Take money or food by force? Create or join a band with similar problems and raid others? Would you kill?

The answers are slightly different for everyone, and be careful about being too glib. "I would do anything for my children" is easy to say. It rings hollow from someone who doesn't even spend that much time with them.

Some more questions, because in our society this brings up emotional sludge and, on many levels, finding your emotional sludge is what glitch hunting is all about. Would you prostitute yourself to feed your children? Would you prostitute your children to feed your children? Would you sell one to feed the others?

People glitch hard on these, and it puzzles me that people who can use words like "kill" so easily freeze on this. I think it is because most can imagine prostitution while murder remains abstract. It is easy to volunteer for something you don't really understand.

You need only look at Thailand or the Philippines to see that parents make these choices even today. When you look at the other choices—robbery, raiding, theft, and murder—you see much of the human condition throughout history. This choice, "What would I do to feed my children?" has driven much of human history . . . and "What will I do to prevent others?" has driven the development of many of the ancient martial arts. They did not arise in a vacuum, but were driven by lives in a world of what seems to us unimaginably casual violence.

It goes deeper as well. Humans are adaptable. The most outrageous situations can come to seem normal. Humans have created societies, philosophies, and religions to justify actions driven by hunger, and things that were originally driven by hunger have, over time, become normal.

If you were willing to kill and rob to feed your children, how long would it take you to become OK with it? To convince yourself what you had to do was not only acceptable, but even noble? People are not so different.

Is this merely a history lesson? Not at all. With a slight tweak, this level of motivation still drives most of the violent crime in the civilized world. Just substitute "addiction" for "starving children."

Without the touchstone of need, most people cannot empathize with what would make addicts kill or steal, burglarize or sell themselves and their children. This thought experiment helps cross that bridge.

If you can imagine what you would do, you can also imagine, and evaluate, what a criminal would do. You need to feed your children: will you attack obviously, from the front, and give plenty of warning? If something happens to you, your children will surely starve . . . if a criminal gets hurt or caught, he will have to deal with withdrawals.

The things that would talk a criminal down are not the psycho-babble ramblings of a therapist, but the things that would talk you down if you had children to feed. They could talk you out of the violence, but only for some money or food, and only if it didn't take too long.

The Predator Mind

Do this: for a day, you will become a bad guy. Go to crowded festivals, parks, and bars, and start looking at the people all around. Who would be easy to take? Who doesn't pay attention? Who leaves the car running when they go somewhere for a quick chore? How many children are alone and unwatched, or supposedly watched by people who are texting away, oblivious?

Can you identify the weak and needy, the ones who would go away with you for just a little attention? The obliviously helpful who would put themselves unwittingly in harm's way and walk with you into a concealed area?

Who would be too proud to scream for help?

In the bully mind, who would be entertaining? Who would scream and beg? What are the weaknesses you would exploit—physical and emotional? If you didn't want to attack the body, how could you attack the identity? People will give away many clues in a few minutes of conversation if you listen.

Who is strong and dangerous? How can you tell? It is not a matter of size but one of will, and you can feel that in people. We all can. Where does it come from? How do you project it?

Where would you attack? What are the blind zones and escape routes? It's not enough to do the crime; you must be able to get away with it. Where are the private areas in public places? Where can you sit and use mirrors and shadows to track everything around you?

For one day, look at the world with the eyes of a predator.

Articulation

Making good decisions is often easier than explaining those decisions. This is especially true in a self-defense situation, where the decision and the action may be made in an instant, and you may need to explain, clearly and logically to police, prosecutors, and a jury, why you had no choice.

That takes practice, but there is more to it.

You make fast decisions all the time. Without reverting to conscious thought you subconsciously take in information, weigh options, and turn right rather than left, or slap your hand over the sudden leak in a hose.

Making rapid decisions is something you already do. Making good rapid decisions is also something you can do, but it takes practice and knowledge. You must have a background of information and experience to base your decisions on.

In a self-defense situation, you *must* understand self-defense law generally and your local jurisdiction's laws in particular. You *must* read them yourself, and you must understand them. You need those facts in your head before your subconscious can make an informed decision.

Generally, if your ego doesn't get involved, you will make good and justified self-defense decisions. Most of the people who claim they have been jailed for self-defense fully participated in bringing on the fight.

That may not matter, though, if you can't explain the decision. "Self-defense" is an affirmative defense. It does not make the underlying crime disappear (e.g., if you have killed someone in self-defense, you have committed the crime of homicide, probably manslaughter). It justifies the crime. It explains it.

You must explain it.

You are unlikely ever to get in enough violent encounters that you can remember them clearly, much less describe them . . . and much less describe them in legalspeak:

After yelling "I'm going to kill you, motherfucker!" the threat then attempted to strike me with his right fist. Because of his size, youth, and strength, he was capable of doing considerable damage and showed intent (threat, attacking), means (size, strength, closed fist), and opportunity (he was well within reach) to be an immediate threat at an assaultive and possibly lethal level. That would have automatically justified focused blows and, given the strength disparity, an impact weapon. I judged that I could evade the blow and push the threat into the wall, which I did, handling the incident a full two levels of force below that which would have been authorized by policy and law.

You won't have an opportunity to dissect many fights if you live a somewhat normal life, but you will have many opportunities to dissect subconscious, faster-than-thought decisions.

Do this: from this point forward, whenever you get a feeling or a hunch, if it is safe to stop and think, stop and think. "Where did that thought come from?"

Your brain processes huge amounts of information all the time. The stuff that makes it to your conscious awareness is a tiny piece and not necessarily the important stuff. Your intuition doesn't trigger from some psychic power. You noticed something, it fit a pattern, and you drew a conclusion.

Figure it out.

In my continual quest to keep some chivalry in the world, I give up my seat on public transportation if a lady is standing. Always. Riding the T in Boston over the summer, in one incident, I didn't. Just instinctively. Why?

The lady was traveling with her husband. She had her hair covered . . . hair covered. Killer shoes? Check. Middle Eastern, then. Had I offered the seat, she wouldn't have been able to take it, not and leave her husband standing. He would have had to take it.

A few moments later, a seat opened up and I saw it play out. He even argued, trying to get her to sit, but she was firm. She would not. He took the vacant seat.

These may seem like very minor things, but your brain works like this constantly.

It may seem that the purpose of this exercise is to get you skilled at explaining subconscious decisions. If you ever need to explain a self-defense decision, you'll definitely need that skill. But that is minor. Like many of the internal workings, this has benefits that have nothing to do with self-defense.

By articulating the causes of your hunches, your conscious mind will come to trust them more. It will trust your intuition. Your intuition, being an old part of the brain and very smart in its own way, will notice this and start throwing more hunches your way.

This exercise becomes a habit and starts to bring different parts of your brain together, slowly dissolving the artificial barrier between conscious and subconscious.

INTERLUDE #4: TRAINING OPEN-ENDED SKILLS

Fighting—not just self-defense, but all forms of human conflict and maybe of human interaction—is enormously complex. It will never be a situation where there is a consistent and obvious answer. It will never be like math or engineering, where tolerances can be measured and one plus one equals two.

As such, it can't be taught the same as a simpler endeavor.

I can throw you some analogies.

You can spend years in classrooms, learning foreign languages. You can have an advanced degree in a foreign language. You may be able to parse a sentence at a level that few native speakers can understand. (Do you know which cases your native language uses? Can you define a gerund or a participle?)

And many have found out, to their consternation, that all that knowledge doesn't automatically translate to conversation. Much less to argument or detailed analysis. Master the basics, learn what you want, but in order to really be fluent in a language, you have to get in there and talk and listen and sometimes argue. You can learn everything about language in a classroom. You only learn to *use* it in uncontrolled interactions with other people.

I don't know a lot about music, so I won't embarrass myself, but jamming strikes me the same way. There are, I hear, some really good technical players who can't jam. That's a separate skill.

Last one, there's a book out there called *Impro: Improvisation and the Theatre*, by Keith Johnstone. All about improvisational theater. It is possibly the best book I've ever read on teaching people to fight. Martial arts, in a way, are very much like acting—stylized, scripted with specific postures that mean specific things—but fighting is very much like improvisation. It is in the moment and comes from your core. Very good actors can't always improvise. Improvisational geniuses sometimes can't stick to a script well enough to be great actors.

And the same mental errors that screw up a fighter screw up an improv actor. Trying to be clever. Trying to remember a good response. Trying to stop actions rather than use them.

One aspect of training that is critical is to get in there and play.

There are problems inherent in that. The essence of this kind of training is inherently not nice. The goal is to get kinetic energy into another body. There is an inverse correlation between effective and safe training. Playing live increases the risk. Playing live forces some safety modifications. Playing live conditions habits, including safety flaws, very deeply. So be careful.

But if you can't play live, no matter how much you know, you can't fight.

To train an open-ended skill you have to play in the milieu. You have to learn to use (and learn to love) the sweaty chaos of slamming and being slammed. Don't fall in love with it. Unlike music or debate, part of the goal in most conflicts is to end them quickly, and extended play can be a bad habit. But to learn to move a body, you must practice moving a body that doesn't want to be moved. To hit a real person, you must learn to strike with power on a moving target at variable distance. The only way to learn about improvised weapons and slamming people into walls or throwing them down stairs is to practice.

C: COMBAT DRILLS

These are the hands-on version of combat, done as realistically and safely as possible—and yes, in combat, self-defense, or martial arts "realistic and safe" is an oxymoron.

What follows trains habits for taking people out. For flipping the switch from day-to-day life to destroying another human being. It will also ingrain just as powerfully each and every safety flaw you construct into the drill.

The best compromise I have found is to work with armor whenever possible. Armor is expensive, and it is not perfect. Most commercial armors severely limit your mobility (with the exception of Tony Blauer's HighGear). All, so far, severely limit your vision . . . which may not be a bad thing, since it accurately mimics the tunnel vision of stress.

None protects you completely. One of the most protective commercial suits available (you can dress a guy in it and throw him down the stairs) did not protect one of our trainers from getting his knee snapped. Except for the bulletman suit, good head protection does not equate with good neck protection: if you know how to hit, you will still injure the neck when the helmet protects the head.

Because of the live, chaotic, and fast nature of these drills, there is a much greater risk of injury than in most other things in this book. Be careful. There is no perfectly safe way to mimic the creation of cripples and corpses.

Takeouts

c

The purpose of this book is not to teach an effective flinch response, but everyone should have one in case of a sudden attack. For more on this, see *Facing Violence* or the works of Tony Blauer.

Whether you do or not, you should train yourself that when attacked, you go on the attack and you do not stop until you are safe. Takeouts are the training method.

Do this: partner A attacks in any way from any angle with any weapon. If he is behind you, you'll probably get hit. Deal with it. The intensity and speed of the attacks should be dependent on the skill and experience of the students. Partner B, the one doing the drill, takes partner A out.

What this means is that as efficiently as possible, fully on the attack (no defense, feinting, or sparring timing), B swarms over A in a flurry. Whatever B trains is on the table—strikes, locks, takedowns . . . As efficiently as possible (which means in as few moves as possible) B makes A "safe." Whether this means down, pushed away, or incapacitated is dependent on the circumstances. Do not think "winning." Refer to the concept of fighting to the goal. Getting away works.

As Loren Christensen said, "There are only so many beats in a fight. I want each of those beats filled with *my* stuff." Once someone triggers your defensive offense, he should never get another action. You should be throwing so much action at him that he freezes.

The OODA loop is a model for how decisions are made in combat, developed by Colonel John Boyd. You must *observe* something, like a sudden pain on the back of your head. Then you *orient*, figuring out what you perceived. "Damn! Someone hit me in the back of the head!" Only then can you *decide* what to do. Then you *act*.

Since your first *observation* is the threat's *act*, when you are defending yourself, you start three steps behind in the process.

More relevant is that if a new *action* happens before you finish the loop, it kicks you back to the first *observe* step. If enough attacks come in (really, if enough information keeps coming in), you will keep bouncing back to *observe*. You will never act. It is a form of freezing that can be triggered and why so many experienced criminals open with a flurry attack.

Training takeouts, first and foremost, is a system to ignore sparring timing where, if you think about it, you wait for an opportunity, you wait for your turn . . . and by the time it is your turn in a flurry, you will probably be finished. Takeouts train you to answer a flurry with an immediate counterflurry.

Over time, it becomes a reflex, and the flurry ceases to freeze you.

The second major aspect of training the takeout is that it induces the OODA freeze in the threat. Bad guys don't usually practice this defensively. They are used to the initial attack working because it usually does. They freeze just like everyone else when the tables are turned.

The third aspect, and the one that is most obvious to martial arts practitioners, is that the takeouts become more efficient with practice. The targeting, power generation, and flow from technique to technique become faster, smoother, and more natural. The ability to read the opponent's body in a glance (and possibly the terrain when you allow environmental fighting with this) and respond to circumstances improves quickly.

Multiman

This can be done in a circle or a line, with or without weapons, and with the environment in play or not. For intelligent practitioners, the environment should always be in play, and if they think of it themselves, they should be praised when they figure out they can run out the door and get away.

The rules are similar to the takeouts drill, except the threats get to keep fighting if they judge that the principal, the defender, has not finished them.

Do this: the threats line up facing the principal (rear, side, or front), or form a circle around him.

One threat attacks. Ten seconds later, whether the first threat is dealt with or not, the instructor sends in a second. Ten seconds later, a third. This goes on for a minute with beginners, usually two minutes or until you run out of threats for advanced practitioners.

Multiman forces efficiency. You deal with one at a time, but if you deal with him half-assed, you will have two, then three, then four, then five . . .

It allows you to work dynamic fighting, the geometry of multiple attackers, and you *will* use environmental fighting, if only by throwing opponents into one another.

There is a variation to this drill, and it carries the potential for a deep inner working. It is not for everybody and not safe. By its nature, it can never be chosen by the student; only the instructor can decide whether to do this or when the time is right. Even then, it can be shattering. I do not do this aspect of the drill—at least I have not done so yet. My mentor has, and he says roughly half of the people cannot deal with what they learn and quit training—and these are students who have spent years in a very serious training environment.

You can speed up the multiman, sending them in at five or three seconds. There is some level at which even the strongest and most skilled practitioner will fail. For this deeper lesson, you don't stop. You pile on more people, take the principal to the ground, and continue. It doesn't stop, not when he taps, not when he uses the safe word that he has been promised will always stop the drill.

The threats do not strike for injury or wrench on locks. They use pressure and pain, no more. The principal is helpless, completely, and *it does not stop*. He will either come to an emotional edge and break or he will pass out. The instructor must watch for that moment.

If the principal passes out and everything was done properly, it is simple anoxia, and he will recover in about twenty seconds. If he does not, it is a medical emergency and needs to be treated as such.

If he breaks emotionally, the instructor must recognize that point and stop the exercise.

Is there a purpose to this? Yes, but it is not for everybody and I repeat, I do not recommend that you do this drill to this level.

There is an important truth: there is no such thing as "safe." No matter who you are or how well you have trained, no matter if you have a Medal of Honor or a world-champion belt, there are levels of violence that can overwhelm you. Not just beat you, but crush you like a bug on a windshield.

The truth is simple, in words. But deep down, no one knows what he will do or who he is when he comes to that level of violence.

Understand this: almost no one has any reason to know who he or she is at that edge. It serves no purpose to know in advance how you deal with imminent death. If you did find out, the experience would probably change it anyway.

It is valuable for some people. Some traditions demand it, for one thing. Some individuals are obsessed with finding out who they truly are at the core. This drill is a big step in that direction, but be warned. You are unlikely to be happy with what you find. Even heroes die screaming for mommy.

Breakthrough

Breakthrough is the simplest and most obvious drill for "fighting to the goal."

Do this: instead of sparring with an opponent or two, the principal must get through a door as quickly as possible. That's all.

The defenders (usually one to three) will react very differently, depending on their instructions. If they have been told to prevent the principal from getting through the door, they will almost always win, but that situation is rare in real violence. The bad guys want to hurt the victim or want something from the victim. If the victim fights, the victim is expected to fight them. A sudden burst of energy toward a different goal almost always has an advantage in surprise and unexpected tactics.

The principal will soon learn that the tactics for fighting and the tactics for escaping or bursting through are very different.

Variations include breaking out of a ring or pushing rapidly through a crowd. The crowd can be focused on the principal or not, making a different dynamic.

Bull in the Ring

This is an awesome drill with a potentially very high injury rate. This was part of the physical test when I first joined the tactical team. We had to discontinue it—as our skill went up, the injury rate did as well. But it was an extraordinary test for learning about instincts.

Do this: in a matted, limited space, place the principal in the center. Two mats making an eight-by-eight-feet square, or a little bigger, twelve by twelve, make a good space. Four threats surround the principal. The threats have kicking shields. The principal is allowed to strike only into the kicking shields . . . and the threats are allowed to hit and slam, but only with the kicking shields. Ideally, everyone is armored.

At the command of "go," the drill begins. If (when) the principal gets knocked down, the threats let him up, not striking again until he at least gets to his knees. He is not allowed to rest, not on the ground, not ever. Nor is the principal allowed to escape the ring. He can try to fight smart and get one of the threats in the center, but the principal can't leave. The drill runs for one minute.

The intense chaos of being knocked around by four strong men is a revelation, and probably the best possible low-injury simulation of being in a riot.

But there is a better reason for this, especially from a recruiting and evaluation standpoint. So far, every person gasses out (runs out of energy) forty-five to fifty seconds into the drill. At that point you see what a recruit's instincts are. When he has nothing left, does he try to curl into a defensive ball? Or is his instinct to fight with nothing left?

In one minute you can get to the combative heart. Former professional football players and reserve Special Forces soldiers have failed at this drill . . . and 120-pound women with no fighting experience have come through like lions.

A note on armor: It's not always for safety. In any drill where immobilization and exhaustion figure, armor often makes people feel claustrophobic, trapped, and unable to breathe. It also limits sound cues and peripheral vision. Often, in stress scenarios, those are training benefits.

The Reception Line

Do this: one student is picked out, and I joyfully announce that he or she has been elected governor. It is now time for the inaugural ball. The principal's first duty is to shake hands with all the people lining up to congratulate him or her—contributors, friends, political allies, and rivals. The student must be nice and friendly, but I warn the principal there is intelligence that someone will try to kill the new governor tonight.

The governor then faces away and one of the other students gets the training knife. All the students are given instructions: be happy, be friendly, shake hands, hug, and then mill around behind the governor. The assassin can attack at any time—while shaking hands, later, after everyone else is done, while the governor is getting a hug . . .

The students cycle through the governor role. At least once, time permitting, there is no assassination attempt, and the whole class gets to take a good hard look at how stilted and weird the body language of someone who is afraid can be. It's educational.

I use the reception-line drill to illustrate a number of things. First and foremost, when done with martial artists, how locked-in we are to finding martial arts solutions to survival problems. The governor almost never runs. Or yells for help, or lets people know a knife is involved. When done in a martial arts studio, most seem to actively avoid using the mirrors all around. Not wanting to cheat? Isn't survival in an ugly situation largely about cheating?

People almost never grab for the weapons on the wall in the dojo.

It's good practice for other things as well—reading a crowd and looking for the giveaways, especially weapon checks. People almost always check concealed-weapon placement when they get tense. Practicing stillness for explosive action even while moving and interacting.

The best, though, came from a man named Peter Breton after he had a day to think about it:

I want to thank you for a great seminar.

You told us that we would get epiphanies about our scenarios later on, and I had a full-fledged refrigerator moment this morning.

You gave me the governor scenario, and I'll tell you honestly, I was disappointed that I got that one. The reason is that some of the other scenarios scared the crap out of me, and I was secretly hoping that I would get something like that. As it was, I had a strong "nothing I could do" feeling . . . and also I felt like I was playing a part on stage.

The truth is, I had hundreds of choices, and I didn't see any of them. I could've badgered you into giving me a chief of security (hey, I'm the governor, right? Where's my fucking chief of security?). I could've announced to the crowd that I had contracted Ebola and wouldn't be able to shake hands with anyone. I could've told you in the anteroom that I personally was going to vomit, or pee myself. Kids who forget their homework are far more inventive than I was.

Instead, I let you set me up to be assassinated, and I went along with it because I knew it was only a fun game. Tactically, that was not a bad plan; I was playing the real game (life) instead of the fake one. But there were better options, and I didn't take them.

When I saw these things, I felt for a moment as if the world opened up for me: "change the rules" became suddenly real, and I thought about other games that I'm afraid to change.

Besides this, I have bruises all along my shoulders from rolling on the floor, and vivid memories of hitting someone with a pool rack. :)

Thanks again,

Peter

Peter was the first to dissect this from a strategic level. Why do I have to play along at all? What are the rules of the game I can change? Who said I have to deal with the world I have been handed?

If you or your students can access this level of insight, whether in self-defense or in life, it is a game changer. Another super power.

Scenario Training

In many ways, scenario training is the culmination of all other training exercises. Done properly, the goal is to get as close to real life as possible, without the physical, psychological, and legal consequences that can attend a real self-defense incident.

At its most basic, scenario training combines armored threats, a realistic, cluttered, and chaotic environment, and a simulated bad situation for the student to test and evaluate.

Doing scenarios is easy. Doing them well is not. And there are a few different ways to do them well.

Each scenario should have a purpose. Sometimes there will be more than one purpose, but don't try to do everything with every scenario. Common goals of scenario training are as follows:

- Stress inoculation. This is the idea that if you are exposed to the chaos and violent action of scenarios, you will be less affected by the circumstances and your own stress hormones when and if a real situation happens. Stress inoculation requires fast, violent scenarios, often with a specific emotional component, like a child victimized or held hostage.

- Facing a specific fear. If a student has revealed that there is a scenario that frightens him or her, the student can safely work it out in a stressful and even fearful environment.

- Working out a glitch. If the instructor feels that a student freezes under stress or may not be able to perform a necessary action under stress, like resort to deadly force, a scenario can be designed to draw that out.

- Confidence. False confidence is deadly. True confidence must arise from competence. Unfortunately, it is easier to instill confidence than competence. If, however, you have a student who is better than she knows, a scenario is a great way to let the truth shine.

- Working judgment in tandem with skills. Many martial artists are taught how to kick and hit without being taught when. The student in the scenario not only must perform, but must also make the proper decisions and explain them properly.

- Breaking training habits. Scenarios are a good place to show that running away and communication, things talked about but not often practiced, are good options.

- Familiarizing with violence dynamics. It takes excellent role-players to get the nuances down, but in many scenarios there should be clues to what is about to happen. As in real life, the person who catches the clues early has more options and can often avoid violence. In any case, the clues also become part of the articulation.

- Familiarizing and practicing legal self-defense. After each scenario the principal will have to explain to a peer jury what he or she did, both tactically and legally. If there are serious misunderstandings of self-defense law, they will come out.

- Articulation. Articulation is severely undertrained. Making a good decision is often far easier than explaining a good decision. The students after each scenario will explain what they did and why.

- Practicing avoidance. Avoidance is the most important aspect of self-defense, yet something that rarely gets more than talk in a training hall or dojo. Avoidance and de-escalation need to be practiced.

- Learn to take a hit and recover. And stick to a plan afterward.

- Pressure testing. You can use scenarios to see if students can execute techniques under the stress of adrenaline and a dynamic situation. More dangerous to the instructor's ego, good scenario training will also show you that some techniques do not work under pressure or have no legal application in the modern world.

- Scenario training is an important step in moving the student beyond technique and into tactics. It is also crucial to developing two of the most important skills for tactical action: the ability to accurately see what is happening and the mental flexibility to improvise under stress.

- Testing. This can be specific or general. A general test is "How do Jimmy's skills hold up under stress?" or "Does Carrie understand self-defense law?" A specific test is designed to find out something: "Will Jerry leave, or is he too proud?" "Will Barb shut it down when she knows it is going bad or wait until her options are gone?"

Safety. Scenarios are high-speed, often high-force training done in a cluttered environment and under stress. People make mistakes. They get adrenalized, and that makes them clumsy. Scenarios can easily become quite dangerous.

You must give a good safety briefing that must include the following points:

- Every person involved—students, role-players, observers, and facilitators—is a safety officer. Anyone who sees something unsafe has the right and the responsibility to stop the scenario.

- A safety word *anyone* can say to stop action.

- All students need to inform the facilitator and role-players of any preexisting injuries.

- Location of first aid kit, identity of assigned medic, and location of nearest emergency room.

- Instructions for how the scenarios will go.

- A physical search to make sure that no one has a live weapon and there are no live weapons in the training area. Anyone who leaves the area should be searched upon return.

- No one under the influence of any mind-altering substance, including prescription medication, is allowed in the training area.

- The safety limitations of the armor.

- The comfort zones of the role-players.

- That people should expect to be hit and knocked down.

- That extremely bad and offensive language will be used—it will be racial, sexual, and personal. It will be designed to push emotional buttons.

- Some of the touching will be inappropriate and might be explicitly sexually aggressive.

- Anyone with injuries needs to tell the instructor and role-players now.
- If anything we've discussed might trigger some psychological issues, talk to the instructor privately. (As an instructor, you will have to make time for this and, ideally, you will have had this talk with each of the students prior to scenario training.)
- There are other aspects of the initial briefing not directly related to safety. Not everyone will get a scary scenario. Do not try to guess what the right solution is. Don't read into the situation. Do not feel that because this is a class you have to do any particular thing. A training weapon in the scenario is to be treated as a real weapon.

Follow through with everything in the safety briefing. Talk to students and search the students and the area. Make sure the training equipment, especially the armor, is in good condition and high quality.

Every armor type has its quirks. My personal set has earholes right over the ears. I've ruptured eardrums with a slap through the helmet. Know your armor and make sure the role-players know the armor. Make sure the students know as much as they need to know, including if the armor can hurt the student (like a face cage that can damage hands if punched).

The role-players should not only have good armor but be skilled fighters. The armor only protects so much. The role-players need to be able to protect themselves and keep their cool.

There is an additional and so far insurmountable safety issue: role-players need to be able to communicate clearly. I haven't been able to do that with a mouth guard in place.

If one of the students has an injury or is otherwise physically vulnerable, you can tailor a scenario that requires judgment instead of hands-on conflict. Generally, though, there should be a risk of violence.

Selecting personnel. Scenario training is hard to do well, and poor-quality scenarios can do far more harm than good. People frequently confuse intensity with reality. This is why the more intense the sparring, the more people feel it is a good test of what works and what doesn't, even if not a single other element of the environment or the encounter mimics a real attack.

So, the first choice in personnel is the scenario designer. This person must have a complete grasp of violence dynamics and force law. If he is relying on fantasy, then scenario training is no more than a LARP (live action role-playing) game.

The second person is the facilitator. The scenario designer is usually the facilitator as well. The facilitator is responsible for matching the scenario with the student (with input from others as needed). Other responsibilities include briefing and debriefing, beginning and ending the scenario, assuming primary responsibility for safety, and signaling to the role-players when to amp up, tone it down, engage, or disengage.

Your facilitator needs to be experienced enough that he doesn't get adrenalized tunnel vision, auditory exclusion, or memory distortion. He or she must understand violence dynamics, force law, articulation, and tactics. The facilitator cannot be ego driven, trying to show off *his* knowledge. He must be able to let the student explain what happened and learn from experience.

The title "role-players" can cover a lot of jobs. In any given scenario, there may be several roles to play or only one. The actors may be important to the scenario or distractions and bystanders. They might be witnesses to groom or people to enlist for help, if the student thinks of it.

It can be difficult to run realistic scenarios with only one suit of armor—the student always knows who to focus on. At the same time, armor for everyone in a big scenario is prohibitively expensive, even for most government agencies. Your armored role-players will take the brunt of any fighting that develops. With good briefings, you can enlist the other students as background, such as all the other people in a crowded, noisy bar when the threat attempts to separate the principal from the herd and talk her into a private place.

The primary role-players must be experienced. They must be good enough at fighting that they can defend themselves, egoless enough that they can let the student win.

A tip from the late Tim Bown, bulletman extraordinaire for all role-players: "In every scenario, before you let them win, you find the one point where you could have finished it. You kind of count coup [see WW5]. That way you don't make the mistake of practicing to lose."

The role-players must be able to act convincingly as bad guys: use the language, the body language, and the tactics of real criminals. This includes everything from the nervous young punk on his first robbery to the experienced professional to the socially skilled rapist. The best are actors as well. They can project whether they are male or female, young or old, with just body language while wearing a helmet and armor.

Role-players also need a certain type of sensitivity. The facilitator will not always be able to predict what students will do. The role-players need to have the awareness and internal sensitivity to tell if a new tactic would have worked. One of the most dangerous mistakes in scenario training is for the instructors (facilitator, designer, and role-players) to lock onto an idea of what they think will work and *only* allow those tactics to succeed. We are there to reward success, including success that is more creative than our own. Recognizing that takes some sensitivity. Acknowledging it takes some humility.

The safety officer (SO) has primary responsibility for the safety of the area and shares responsibility for safely conducting the scenario. He or she maintains and inspects all equipment, makes sure all safety equipment is properly worn, and pat searches anyone entering the training area.

Before scenarios the SO goes over the area, looking for any hazards. Exposed nails, shelves at inconvenient heights, broken glass, areas of bad footing, or hidden steps. Anything that might prove dangerous. The SO makes the call on if the hazard should be removed or barricaded, marked, noted, or ignored.

Items with high risk and no training value should be removed when practical. Broken glass on the floor may add to the ambience, but it can only injure and adds no value to the training. If removal is not possible, the hazard should be barricaded—blocked off by something strong enough that the role-players will not just crash into the hazard.

If that is not practical, the hazard or certain areas of the training venue can be marked off limits. Bright tape, like crime-scene tape, or orange traffic cones are a decent choice.

In certain circumstances I will have a hazard pointed out to all participants but left in play. "Notice that there is a slight step here between the dance floor and the stage. Be careful, but if it is appropriate, this is one of the things I want you to think about using."

That is specialized, something you do with experienced fighters that you are trying to get to polish specific awareness skills.

Sometimes the decision is made to ignore the hazard. Remember that part of conducting a good scenario is to maximize the perceived danger while lowering the actual danger. Some things look dangerous but are big and obvious. No one misses those. When we do scenarios at Chris's cabinetry shop in Ontario, you don't have to warn people about the table saw.

The peer jury. The remaining personnel necessary to make scenario training work is everyone else. All the other students and observers. There is a little debate here. Some trainers keep the scenarios secret with no witnesses and run everyone through the same scenario.

If you have a limited number of scenarios, that is efficient, but there are a few problems. If ten people are going through the same scenario out of sight of one another, 90 percent of the time will be spent waiting. The teachers won't notice that—they'll be busy—but the students will be twiddling their thumbs.

Students learn from watching other students. If the students do not watch others, they will get exposed to only one concept in a training session. They will get some stress inoculation and might pick up a few things, but watching a dozen scenarios where slightly different things are important allows for a dozen complex learning opportunities.

Witnesses, especially people you know, add another level of stress, a form of performance anxiety. More stress is good. With no student witnesses, no peer jury, the student running through the scenario may not recognize his own stress-fueled memory distortion. He may remember things far more heroically than they happened and will choose not to believe the facilitator.

Video is a good option, if you have the resources. It makes very clear what actually happened, and it leaves little room for heroic memory. It does, however, require more resources, including personnel. There are always privacy issues. No one should be allowed to record a scenario session unless you have specific releases from all participants.

After each scenario, the student explains her actions, both from tactical and legal standpoints, to the other students. The mistakes and missed opportunities tend to be obvious. The facilitator must monitor that the peer jury input doesn't get too weird. When you ask people for input, they tend to give you input, and when there isn't that much useful to say they tend to get very speculative—read: weird.

Designing scenarios. Designing good scenarios is actually not that hard. Just remember to keep them realistic, make them appropriate to the student, and have them serve a purpose.

The easiest way to create realistic scenarios is to look at crime dynamics and crime statistics and to remember times when you were nervous or thought a situation could have gone bad. If there has been a group attack in a parking garage, find out what you can, and then talk with your role-players about setting it up: three young men coming up the stairs talking and laughing see a potential victim and suddenly go silent and spread out . . . There are lots of clues in that little sentence.

Looking at times that might have gone bad, what about aggressive panhandlers or mentally disturbed people who either remember the student or think they do? At what point is excessive familiarity dangerous?

Appropriate to the student. If you have a three-hundred-pound football player who moves well, he's not going to be mugged (without a gun and from a safe distance) or randomly attacked from ambush. The most intense scenarios are most likely to happen to the smaller and weaker, and the students know this. The three-hundred-pounder will get a lot of monkey dance–style challenges that are no-win situations for him. If he wins physically, he's the bad guy just because of his size. He needs to understand de-escalation and, if that fails, articulation and witness preparation.

Serving a purpose. I use three carjacking scenarios and play them consecutively with different students. The first is straightforward: a carjacking at gunpoint while the vehicle is stopped. In the second scenario the student's baby is in a car seat in the vehicle. In the third version there is no child, but the newspaper ran an article that morning on three carjackings in this area where the driver was executed after giving up the keys. Those three scenarios show how special knowledge or special circumstances change decisions.

In the parking garage scenario above, I want the students to be able to articulate that not only was the spreading out of the three teenagers a direct threat, but the fact that they went silent as they did it was good evidence this was not their first time. It was an experienced team.

As you design your scenarios, look at the list of purposes and see which, specifically, the scenario fulfills.

If you are dealing with specialized groups (cops or women's self-defense or people learning a specific weapon, like an expanding baton or firearms), there is often a much narrower range of purposes. With cops, the scenarios are usually to determine if they can appropriately engage at the right level of force and whether they can articulate it. Almost every scenario will be aimed at one of those two things. With women's self-defense, most of the scenarios are either designed to show critical decision points (when things can be stopped from going bad) or to see if the students have given themselves permission to really unload on a threat. With weapons groups, part of it is knowing how to use the weapon, but the primary purposes are demonstrating the judgment of when *not* to use the weapon and articulating the reasons to a jury when you must use the weapon.

Selecting a location. I like running scenarios in nightclubs and bars, places where bad stuff tends to happen. You can do carjacking drills in a vehicle parked on the street. (Strangely enough, most cruising patrol cars see a guy using the same training armor they train with surrounded by an audience of twenty to thirty people and they don't get excited.)

You can also create a modular training area, if you have access, using tarps and rope to change the shape of walls and padding everything up. It can be safer, and if you are doing a lot of scenarios in the same area, it is probably cost effective.

You can do scenarios almost anywhere you can get permission to do them. The one place I don't recommend is a training hall or dojo, for three reasons.

First, there will almost always be some reality concessions made. Some are purely practical: boots tear up mats and play hell with hardwood floors, but the second people try to do scenarios barefoot, it starts to feel unreal. If the concessions demanded are less practical, such as bowing, it can compound the feeling.

The second is related. Students have a specific mind-set associated with the places they train. It doesn't matter if they are emulating modern Spetsnaz or ancient Japanese warriors; they get into the mind-set of what they are supposed to do as martial artists, not what they need to do to survive. Changing to a real-world location really helps people break patterns they have developed in training.

Third, I want them to get dirty. To roll on filthy concrete, get messy and sweaty, dodge obstacles, and use obstructions and debris for weapons. Fights happen in the world, and much of the world, especially where bad stuff happens, is an amazingly messy place. Students need to not only get used to that but to also exploit it.

The flow of training—these instructions are written for the facilitator:

1. If possible, meet with each student and, when you can, meet with the student's instructor. Ask the instructor what the student needs. Assign the students to a scenario on your list. There is a rhythm to it. Don't assign all the harsh scenarios at the beginning or the end of the day. Keep them unpredictable. Especially early in the day, you want the students to see what a wide variety of issues will be involved. It's good to have the role-players at these meetings as well.

2. Give the safety briefing.

3. Tell which student(s) will be in the first scenario.

4. Brief the role-players. They should already be familiar with the scenario. Give them special instruction, such as whether the student

has an injury to be aware of, whether you want this scenario extra intense, or if you are worried about this student's power or control.

5. Brief the student. This is usually done in the ready area outside the main scenario area. The briefing should have the minimum necessary information: "You are going to an all-night convenience store around 0200. When you step through into the training area, you have opened the door." You will also at this time tell the student anything you are simulating: "The big cardboard box is the counter. The guy in the blue shirt is the clerk." You will also tell the student the role of the other students: "The other students are not there. You can't see them."

6. If necessary, brief the other students. Sometimes they will have to play bystanders, corpses, or witnesses. Assume they are not experienced role-players and be explicit on whether they should get involved and how much they are allowed to do.

7. Make sure that everyone who needs safety equipment has it on properly.

8. Conduct the scenario. The commands I use are "Start scenario!" "End scenario!" and a special word that indicates a safety problem and an immediate freeze. I also use hand signals with the role-players: hand raising up, palm to sky, means increase the intensity, becoming meaner and more belligerent. Palm down, lowering like I'm patting a dog, means decrease intensity. Hand coming toward my chest means close distance on the student. Hand pushing away is back off. Fingers across throat: It's over. Retreat or surrender or walk away.

9. End the scenario.

10. Debrief

Debriefing is probably the most important skill in scenario training. A scenario is an intense experience, but if it isn't processed, that is all it is. A jumbled sense of intense impressions in a stew of stress hormones. The debriefing is needed partially to wring out the lessons but largely to process the experience.

It should be simple, and the student should do most of the talking. I usually start with, "OK, Chris. What did you see? What did you do?"

Then sit back and let Chris tell the story. What she saw, what she did, and why. The tactics always come first because it is more natural for most people, closer to the way that they think.

Generally, if the facilitator has questions or wants to bring something up, he should ask the student: "Chris, when did you know it was going to go bad? Why didn't you act right then?" Or ask the peer jury.

There will be things the peer jury saw and heard that the principal did not. This is where the facilitator can talk briefly about the sensory distortions under stress. There will be clues built in that most will miss, such as after a *stranger* assault. "How many heard him say, 'Bitch, I've had all I'm going to take from you!'? What did that indicate? Does that go into your articulation?"

After the tactics, you want the student to explain her actions in accordance with self-defense law. With practice, this should be very specific, but you will have to lead the first few. The students should explicitly explain the following:

- how they knew the threat had the intent, means, and opportunity to be an immediate threat;
- what level of threat existed (none, passive, active, assaultive, deadly);
- any relevant factors or circumstances;
- if force was used, why nothing else would work (preclusion); and
- what level of force she could have legally justified and what level of force she in fact used.

You will find, and the students will find, that even under stress, most of their force decisions are good, but a good decision can be torpedoed by a bad explanation. Articulation takes practice. Lots of practice.

Common Problems in Scenario Training

- Too many scenarios for each student. Realistically, most male students burn out of adrenaline after one rough scenario and aren't ready to feel those effects again for some time. Women tend to get adrenalized after their scenarios are over. It's biological.

- If you put a student through too many scenarios, he goes into a game mind-set and stops treating the scenario with respect. This is different for police and military units, who will train the scenario again and again, rehearsing for tactical effect. Professionals do not do scenarios for the same reasons that most civilians do.

- Weirdness creep: For the students, each scenario is new and exciting. For the facilitator, designer, and role-players, they may have repeated each one hundreds of times and started to find them boring. There is a tendency to "spice up" scenarios you have done many times. You need to fight this. Keep the scenarios realistic, appropriate, and purposeful. Challenging for the student, not fun and challenging for you . . . or you will wind up with scenarios featuring robot pirates, aliens, and intelligent monkeys.

- Defining the win. There is a philosophy out there that students must be "programmed for success" that every scenario should end with a clear win for the student. All I can say is that I am aware of exactly zero high-end teams that train that way. We learn our lessons via mistakes, and we only improve if we learn.

> If everything goes well in training, it's not training. It's masturbation.

- Defining the win 2: Already touched on, but insecure trainers want the students to do what the trainer would have done. The students aren't you, and they may come up with superior options. Acknowledge and praise anyone who can end a scenario with less force than you would have used.

- Complete student meltdown. Sometimes you will run a scenario that triggers an extreme emotional response in the student. The first step is for the role-player to transition to coach. While still actively engaged, the role-player changes his verbal responses to, "Fight me. You can do this. Take me out." The other students can also shout encouragement. I usually don't encourage that—when bad things happen, you will be profoundly alone and you need to find motivation internally—but in this instance it is better than giving up. If all else fails, the facilitator ends the scenario. In debriefing it is critical to frame this as a learning opportunity, not a failure.

Everyone has a breaking point. This student has found a breaking point. Just finding it changes it. What was the lesson, what was learned, where did the inaction come from, and what internal work is necessary to understand and change the breaking point?

- Most student failures are not problems; they are learning opportunities.

Woofing and super-woofing. "Woofing" is when a bad guy (or self-defense instructor) tries to get you to freak out with his words and body language. He can act loud and scary or quiet and coldly vicious. The words will be chosen to hit your buttons and nothing is off the table. In this world there are no polite euphemisms. Murderers will say "nigger" if they want to.

If you were raised to consider "bitch" as a very mean thing to say to a woman, it's about time you learned that "cunt stain," sometimes shortened to just "stain," is more common in this world.

The words and threats a bad guy uses are designed to make you freeze. You might freeze for a second of shock ("What was that?"), or summoning indignation ("That was so rude! I can't believe it!"), or just in pure terror ("If he said that, what is he willing to *do*?"). If you freeze, for those seconds you will be helpless. The threat knows this, and he counts on it.

Woofing "light" is just the generic way any threat would talk, combined with violating personal space, maybe some touching, like a shove . . . monkey-dance stuff. The students get to deal with some emotion, some confusion, deciding when acting would be legal.

It actually doesn't take much to give the students a taste.

In super-woofing you bring the subject to a mental edge—real fear, real humiliation, and helplessness. It usually takes extensive knowledge of the student's history, fears, and weaknesses. There are ways to bring it out in almost anyone, but those methods have a severe psychological risk and won't be discussed here.

Super-woofing dredges up a lot of shit. The advantage is that it brings some things out that are hidden—fears, limitations, stuff like that. Real woofing increases self-doubt, but it does so by decreasing self-deception.

It is also rarely necessary or even beneficial to take people this far. Only a very few people have any need to know their breaking point or even that they have one. Life is far more comfortable without some knowledge.

Most of the alternatives are compromises, trying to get the benefits of super-woofing without the dangerous side effects. It doesn't work that well because the dangerous side effects are really the point. Briefing beforehand or a safe word, for instance, dilutes the fear, and fear is one of the points.

To maximize the effects of super-woofing, you let the subjects hit rock bottom and then fight back out. There are three problems with that. First, it takes a hell of a lot of acting skill to convince an intelligent person she legitimately fought out (because she didn't . . . I had to deliberately leave a chance). Second, some can't recover and make themselves fight—and that is a horrible thing to find out about yourself. Third, if they do dig down deep and fight, I will almost certainly be injured. Probably not too seriously—I'm pretty experienced at taking care of myself in close quarters—but if anyone really lets loose, I can be hurt despite armor.

Briefing afterward, especially with a group of close friends, will help a lot.

As bad as a real woof can be for the subject, it can be almost as bad to watch. Especially if you really care.

Scenario training has dangers beyond the safety concerns mentioned above.

- Intensity is easily mistaken for truth. Good scenario training, especially with effective woofing, will change the relationship with the instructor. If the instructor plays a genuine, intense bad guy, the students will sometimes start to think that this is the "real" person.

  o The best solution is to use outsiders to play the bad guy. Second best is for the students to see you do a ritual (meditation) going into and coming out of the role.

- Failure. Sometimes—often, actually—in an intense scenario a skilled martial artist or person with an identity as some kind of hero or protector will fail utterly. Or they will succeed, but they will do so like a normal person in a chaotic mess of uncontrolled action and fear. Very few people live up to their expectations in scenarios or real life. For some, when it has become an identity, it can be pretty devastating.

  ○ Solution: This has to be handled in debriefing. No plan survives first contact, and damn few identities survive going to the edge. Awesome. Now that the false expectations are out of the way, we can start training to become real-world heroes.

- Dissatisfaction with current training. Even experienced martial artists rarely display recognizable skill in a scenario. (They do use their skills, actually, but most can't see the deep principles that did come out in the chaos. They are looking for clean technique.) Some decide what they have learned, no matter what it is, is crap. They quit or start looking for something else. Especially if you are the instructor, you won't see this coming because only the most confident of students will state their dissatisfaction with your training to your face. Look for the guy who gets quiet and leaves early. Usually it was one of the better students as well.

  ○ The solution is two pronged: first and foremost in the briefing before training and in discussions leading up to scenario training, emphasize that this will be a first taste of chaos. With the jury watching it will be like the first time asking someone on a date or the first black belt test. Second, in debriefing, have the students break down what surprised them, what they weren't ready for, and brainstorm ways to practice. Here's a big hint: even people who train specifically in reality-based systems tend to suck in their first scenarios.

- Not doing what you think you are doing. Some things that seem like good ideas can have disastrous consequences. If, for example, you choose to woof by having role-players verbally abuse your students while your students just listen, are you getting the students used to the verbal abuse? Or are you accidentally conditioning them to do nothing when someone makes threats and invades their personal space?

- ○ Solution: Always check any drill for the flaw. Safety flaws have already been mentioned, but look for strategic and tactical flaws as well. It is always a good idea to get someone you trust to check your ideas. Many of our best ideas fall into our own blind spots. You need a friend (or an honorable enemy) to show you what you cannot see.

- Ignorant scenarios are unforgivable. The scenarios are where you as an instructor will imprint what a student is to see, do, and say. Scenarios cannot be about your ego, and they cannot be based on guesswork about how bad things happen. The brain treats information received in intense circumstances as more valid.

  - ○ Solution: Don't guess. Whenever possible, base your scenarios on real incidents.

"Why did you quit?" I asked.

"You shot me."

"No, I didn't. I pointed a plastic gun at you and said, 'Bang, bang.' You didn't feel a bullet tear through your heart. For that matter, if you had felt a bullet tear through your heart, that means you're still conscious, and you have about ten seconds to take me with you.

"Everybody listen up: you aren't dead unless I say you're dead. Some piece-of-shit criminal took ten rounds and still killed one officer and almost beat another to death. If he can take ten to the chest and head and fight on, so can you.

"We *do not* practice dying in here. None of you have my permission to die. You aren't allowed to die in training, and you aren't allowed to die in the streets."

WW: WORLD WORK

Some drills have to be executed in the real world, or at least with a group of people.

The Clothespin Game

This one is fun and appropriate even for children. It could be done in a training hall, but I was introduced to it in a challenge course facilitator training program and the outdoors works for me, as will any place where you have a group of friends or training companions together.

The game requires a clothespin and a group. It can be done while you are doing something else—out hiking, doing a survival class, running through scenarios.

Do this: early in the day, before the first meeting or briefing, when people start to show up, you clip the clothespin to one of the people. This shouldn't be hard. If you can't attach a clothespin to one of a group of unsuspecting people without being caught, you probably aren't ready for this game.

After that you announce, "One of you has a clothespin attached to your clothes. That person has been assassinated."

Then you explain how the game works. If you find the clothespin on yourself, you can get rid of it by putting it on someone else. If you catch someone trying to pin you, that person can't try on you again and, if you want, you can announce to the rest of the crowd who to watch. It is in your own best interest not to let people know if you find the clothespin and not to tell the person who is currently pinned.

At the end of a designated time—half hour, hour, or whenever the group leader feels like it—"It's time. Who has the clothespin?"

Whoever has the clothespin has been assassinated and must sing a song to the assembled group.

The primary purpose of the drill is obvious. To succeed you must be extremely alert to who is entering your space. Further, you are playing this game while doing something else—nature photography or building shelters or rock climbing or shopping. That is a different type of awareness, a hindbrain–forebrain link where most of your mind is concentrating on the task at hand while the rest keeps watch.

The secondary benefit is in public singing. Some people rate public speaking as their greatest fear. In my experience, the adrenaline from performing tastes like the adrenaline from interpersonal conflict. You don't want to sing in public and make a fool of yourself. I can guarantee you won't want to fight and take a chance on being killed or crippled. Both are things that, on a very deep level, you don't want to do. Both are things you must force yourself to do.

Singing is a major step in using will to overcome the freeze.

Ten New Things

We get very complacent, especially about places we know well. Imagine a clock on your home or office wall, one that has been hanging there forever. Who made it? The manufacturer is probably printed right on the face. Is the second hand red or black? Are the numbers in Arabic or Roman numerals? Does the clock have a border? What color?

That's something you see every day.

Do this: ten new things is simply a practice, every so often, to look at a place you know well and notice ten new things about it. Your bedroom. The walk from your car to where you spend your day.

You can do this with things you do every day as well, and sometimes that involves a little research: Why aren't keyboards set up alphabetically? Is there a logic to the QWERTY keyboard? (There is, by the way, and it is a stupid logic.) How do keys and locks work?

In your martial practice you can go as deep or broad into detail, and sometimes you find out things you never expected . . . like that the differences in slashing in Filipino, Japanese, and European systems may have had much more to do with blade construction than with efficiency of motion.

Then, of course, you can apply it to people you know. I guarantee you can find out ten or a hundred new things about people you have spent your whole life with. Ask some questions. Listen.

Stalking

Stalking is one of the oldest skills of mankind. It predates mankind. Cats do it. Dinosaurs probably did it. It is truly a fusion of skills that span awareness, thought, and motion.

Do this: practice the primary skills of moving silently, moving slowly, staying concealed, blending, and working the psychology of your prey.

Moving silently requires good balance, smooth coordination, and sensitivity. Walking, each foot feels the ground before it is planted and then the weight *rolls* onto the foot. If there is something under the foot that might snap, no weight can go on that part of the foot. Things that might rustle, like leaves, are compressed slowly.

Crawling requires more patience and sensitivity, also some strength. The hands move up a bit in front of your head. In the dark, they become your antennas. The feet flex forward so the toes can grip. Slowly, the hands and feet press and you go forward the distance your foot can support your weight from flexed to extended.

Moving slowly fools the eye. Peripheral vision is drawn to motion. There is a threshold past which motion is slow enough that it doesn't draw the eye. For an extreme balance and leg-strength exercise, cross a room taking a full minute to execute each step. Especially challenging when you have to step over noisy obstacles.

Staying concealed can get into a lot of camouflage and face paint. Mud works fine. Do not contrast with your background (e.g., try not to stand in front of dark objects while wearing light colors). Try to conform to the shapes around you, which means break up your shape: hunch, twist, and make rounded contours. Be especially careful not to directly show eyes or teeth. A smiling face stands out because we are conditioned to recognize those features.

Blending is a slightly more complex skill. In city stalking, it is a matter of not standing out. Dress appropriately for the area and time, as well as your age. A big part of blending and stalking in a city is to move naturally. Beginning stalkers go into a very visible mode when they go on the hunt. Any difference in the expected, any pattern disruption, draws the eye. Something as simple as graceful athletic movement, on a street full of commuters, will be noticed. If you naturally walk smoothly, in a city you will have to match the uncoordinated jerkiness all around you.

That same jerkiness will be noticed by animals. Smooth is less visible to them.

Whatever you are stalking—man or deer or housecat—will have a specific psychology. Most people are oblivious unless they have a reason to be paranoid. You can follow them all day, sometimes spend a full minute in touching distance in a crowd, and they are unlikely to remember or notice you . . . but draw attention even once, and they will start looking for patterns and motives and will create a terrifying stalker/slasher story in their imagination.

Deer are a prey species and live in constant fear, and you smell, move, and have eyes like a predator. You can overcome a deer's natural inclinations (with corn or salt or in some national parks), but those are not the ones to stalk. The deer will move casually away if it notices you, unless startled, not wanting to draw attention with fast motion. Interestingly, you can sometimes get quite close by pretending to be absorbed in something else. A wildlife photographer once told me that he got such good pictures by pretending to search for his wallet until he was close enough.

Does a moose know what a wallet is? No, but a moose can tell when he is not the focus of attention.

The test, the challenge, the constant exercise is to try to stalk a wild animal. To see how close you can get to a rabbit or a deer. You will continuously improve.

Escape and Evasion   WW4

This is a skill that must become a habit. You will probably not have to run from a threat very often in your adult life, but running intelligently is a skill, and laying the groundwork early can make all the difference.

Do this: wherever you are right this second, name the fastest way out. What is your first backup option? Second?

Are there places you could hide with a few seconds' notice? Do those places have at least two easy escape routes if you get found? Obviously, the threat who finds you will be in one of the escape routes.

What in your immediate area could stop a handgun bullet? A rifle bullet?

Of the people nearby, who would panic? Who would follow your lead? (And this might be a problem: if escape and evasion become a habit, you will likely be the only one with a plan if things go bad. That kind of puts you in a leadership position. Sorry, pal.)

In all the places where you spend a lot of time, you should know all the exits and where they lead. You should also know which approach is most likely for a typical threat (think enraged former employee, not a tactical team) and not count on that as part of your escape route.

Which windows could be broken and, if you are on a higher floor, how would you negotiate the drop? Would it even be possible? Which walls and doors could be smashed or cut through and how long would it take?

Where would be a safe place to stop running? Far enough away to be safe, out of range of gunshot from the likely threat, access to communication and help, and further escape routes just in case.

For your family, have you gone over how to get out of the house? Where to meet if you get separated in a mall?

For that matter, and tying into the "Ten Things" (WW2), what were your children wearing this morning when they left for school? If they didn't arrive, what description would you give the police?

It becomes an exercise in places you know. Ideally, a drill and a habit in places you just pass through. How do I get off the street right now? Can I run my car off the road here and keep going? Where are the nearest police stations and hospitals?

Every time you get on a plane, read the damn little card with instructions. The plane probably won't crash, but if it does, almost everyone will panic. If you are lucky enough not to panic, it might be kind of nice to know how to open the emergency doors rather than count on there being enough light and little enough smoke to read the instructions at the time.

Two children's games are ideal for developing this skill: tag and hide 'n' seek. If you're too old to play them or too dignified or stuck up, I'm sorry. At least encourage your children to play them and be creative.

Counting Coup

Counting coup was a Plains Indian tradition. Either through stalking or in battle, young men would show their courage by touching an enemy. It had many of the skills of combat with none of the body count. This version is a form of urban stalking, and you will find that threats, especially young men (a.k.a. delinquents), play it all the time. It shows all the skill of mugging but without the legal consequences.

Do this: the idea is to get to perfect range on a target, either without the target being aware or with the target fully aware but doing nothing about it.

Public places, especially crowded ones, are easy. You pick a target and drift or stalk over within range. Without a crowd it is far more difficult, and thus more challenging. If you are ready, see how long you can stay undetected in the striking range.

Counting coup on a fully aware target is more a psychological game than a physical one. It has dangerous psychic elements in it that need to be addressed as safety issues.

To deliberately move into someone's personal space with his knowledge but without permission is an insult. It is punking. In some places and subcultures, if you misjudge, you will have to be ready to defend yourself, and it will not be self-defense because you started it.

More importantly, if someone has a weak ego and is looking for validation, punking people can be addictive. I've said don't practice losing and don't practice missing because you will do it under stress. Now I'm saying, "Don't practice being an asshole because you will become one." And not just under stress either.

You should do it once or twice, partially to notice your own internal resistance to breaking such a cultural taboo and also so that you notice how few people set boundaries in any way. They expect you to respond to the taboo.

See how that works in an assault? Breaking a social taboo indicates that most social controls are off the table for the threat . . . and yet victims expect the social controls to kick in any second. Don't count on it.

Another layer, common among criminals who don't have an immediate need for anything but want to stay in practice, is *forcing*. Forcing is used here the way a magician uses it. There is no coercion or violence or threat. You pick a card, and the card you pick was chosen for you long ago. You were, without being aware of it, forced to choose a preordained card.

In counting coup, forcing is when you do not approach the target but set things up so the target approaches you. Look at young men standing too close to a concession stand or slightly crowding an aisle, forcing people, particularly young women, to brush as they pass. Contact. Counting coup.

There are multiple values in this drill. The stalking practice not only lets you move and think as a predator, but the blending will also help keep you off the predator's radar. You will likely uncover some of your own social conditioning. Far more people will read this description than will actually play the game. And you will also notice how powerful social conditioning is in others. Many will not see you or will convince themselves that your stalking behavior doesn't mean anything. Real predators rely on that denial.

Victims are good people. They don't want to draw attention or make scenes. So they don't set boundaries, and they do put themselves in vulnerable positions.

Say No

This is a stand-in for breaking a lot of social conditioning. Just as physically you may have to respond with decisive action, decisive talk might well prevent things from escalating to force in the first place.

But it takes practice.

Boundary setting is saying, "This far and no farther." It is never a negotiation or a suggestion. A boundary is an incontrovertible fact, and it must be so in your mind and voice. It must have penalties for transgression. If it does not, if a threat violates your boundaries and you do nothing, he will know that none of your boundaries are real.

No. "No" is a complete sentence. Say "no." Say it loud. Too shy? Good to know. Get over it. My editor is having grammar conniptions right now. "It is not a complete sentence. We need a subject and a verb, and sometimes the subject—you—is implied."

Here's the deal: "No" plus any explanation is a *negotiation*. The second it becomes a negotiation, it ceases to be a "no." Criminals and salespeople and anyone who has a stake in manipulating your boundaries know this. If you treat your boundaries as anything other than complete and incontrovertible sentences, they are not boundaries.

Do this: when you don't want to do something and there is no relationship (telemarketers, a stranger offering you a drink in a bar, someone asking you to sign a petition you don't believe in), say, "No."

That's easy. Here's the hard part. Don't explain yourself. No one except you and possibly some friends ever need to know what you are thinking. Don't try to soften it with a "sorry" or an excuse. You did not initiate this contact, and there is no relationship to preserve. Conversation creates relationship. That's something you don't want, especially with a predator.

This will be very hard for most people. Some never get comfortable with it, but it is a critical skill and an act of will.

If the other person tries to establish a conversation/relationship, whether it is the signature seeker saying, "But don't you care about the . . ." or the slimeball in the lounge saying, "Oh, baby, don't be like that . . ." shut it down. "No!" Again. Louder. Deliberately drawing attention.

Eeek! Attention! People will think I'm rude. I'd better not. I don't want people to think . . .

Bad guys count on this thought process. It keeps you meek and predictable. Get this through your head: if you can't make yourself say "no," you won't be able to make yourself fight. Bad guys not only know this about you better than you do, they depend on it.

That is enough. Louder, stronger, but most people won't push past the second "no." They will say some mean shit when they walk away. So what?

The only thing to be concerned with is someone who ignores the second "no" and tries to get closer. Your body will read the approach as a physical threat, which it is. The bad guy will be counting on you to go social.

Most of our experience with conflict has been social conflict. When someone gets really mad and can hurt us (bosses, financially, and parents usually, physically), we tend to apologize and excuse what we've done.

Bad guys know this and expect your reaction to an immediate threat to be social. If you go that route, he has invaded your space, disregarded your "no," and is now completely confident that your boundaries are nonexistent. He owns you.

When and if someone closes after you have set a boundary, prepare to defend that boundary. That doesn't always mean fight, but if there are no witnesses and someone gets close after being told not to, you are likely dealing with a predator. Be fully prepared to do harm in that case.

For the most part, though, boundaries are enforced socially. When someone closes after a "no," the yell becomes, "I told you to back off, you pervert!" and all eyes turn to the scene. Bringing attention is a consequence.

In other circumstances, there are acknowledged channels for enforcing boundaries, such as reporting crimes or violations to the proper authorities.

The boundary-setting progression, in four steps:

Set the boundary. "No," or, "Back off!" for instance.

Restate the boundary, with emphasis: "I said *no!*" or, "*Back off!*"

Boundary+consequences: "Do X now" (X=leave, back off), or I will Y." (Y=tell the boss, call the police, yell, shoot you.)

None of these steps is ever repeated. This is never a conversation. Once the consequences are stated, you must follow through.

Remember—there are situations where you do not have the time to talk and situations where talking will not work. If you find yourself there, be ready to go physical immediately.

Dog Handling

Almost all preventable conflict is about dominance, territories, or enforcing expected behaviors. It is social. Many of the tactics that work socially will not work on predators, and most of what works on predators is illegal or inappropriate for social violence.

Humans are social primates. We get along after a fashion, with constant friction and usually doubt and emotional turmoil.

Dogs are pack animals. They are more social than humans, and without the angst or doubt. That makes them a perfect place to really see pack dynamics.

I'm not sure what follows will help you if you have never been exposed to dogs. If you were raised with several dogs, you know this stuff.

Do this: find someone who trains dogs and pick up some good books on obedience training. *Not* the bullshit books on using treats to train. It's a good tactic for training but gives little or no insight on pack dynamics. Domestically and in the wild, dogs do not use food treats to maintain the social order.

This is hard to describe as a drill, do *this* and you will learn *that*. It is a matter of exposure and observation followed by interaction and more observation.

These are all lessons that apply directly to people:

Older dogs do not play dominance games with puppies. Small dogs pick fights with big dogs, but almost never do big dogs pick fights with small dogs—though they sometimes just kill them. Dogs do not fight dogs the way they attack squirrels or cats.

Dogs respond poorly to uncoordinated people. Slow, smooth movement and slow, smooth speech is comforting for dogs. It is comforting for terrified or very angry people as well. As people get more emotional, their limbic systems start to override their forebrains, and earlier, animalistic behaviors come out.

Dogs have a specific threat display they use on people and other dogs, but not on squirrels. (If someone closes to attack without a threat display first, what does that mean?)

There are specific submission postures and play postures as well, and there are ways to evoke those responses.

Alphas do not get agitated when they are secure. Fighting for status is always a sign of insecurity with the status. A leader on his way down thinks he is stronger being loud and aggressive, but it is a sure sign of imminent failure.

When a new dog comes in, everybody sniffs butts. "Hey, who are you? Where ya from? What'd you do? You hate squirrels too?" A dog that doesn't reciprocate or acts afraid is ostracized. Possibly driven away. Maybe hurt.

The first part is observing the behaviors and figuring out what they mean. It is not hard. We are social animals, not as clear or complete as a pack at that level, but close enough that all of these behaviors make sense.

The second part is to insert yourself into a dog's world. How do you approach a strange dog, especially one that is not well socialized or is frightened? When you can do that reliably, you will have a huge edge in dealing with emotionally disturbed people. When you can recognize when it is *not* safe to approach a scared dog, that wisdom applies to people as well.

When you know how to dominate a Rottweiler, especially without touching him, you will have the body language that people naturally respect as well. When you can mix with a group of strange dogs and not upset the balance of power or make enemies, you will have a relatively easy time working with different cultures, even with a language barrier.

One note: don't get caught up in the "alpha male" bullshit. Most of what is out there for the public seems to be a blend of old studies on wolves, old studies on chimps that borrowed some of the terminology, poorly understood by laymen with an agenda and then applied to people. Garbage in, garbage out is one thing. Misunderstood garbage in is worse.

Want to be a human alpha? Do you want that kind of respect? A human alpha has more resources and uses those resources to help others.

If you haven't accumulated anything that counts as a resource, like skill, wisdom, strength, or wealth, you are effectively a child, dependent on others. If you have accumulated resources and use them just for your own benefit, you're a dick. Have resources and help others, you're an alpha. That doesn't mean you're necessarily a leader or a boss, but you will be worthy of respect.

Global Awareness   WW8

Kasey Keckeisen is a good friend, a superior martial artist, and a SWAT operative, leader, and trainer. Several of us have done experiments and exercises like his Kato-Cato, but few have written about it so well. And so with his permission:

I did an experiment thirteen years ago that helped me start to understand some concepts about how violence happens in the world and how to adjust training methods to compensate for the differences.

I called it the Kato-Cato experiment because it happened in Mankato University and it reminded me of Cato from the *Pink Panther* movies.

Around 1997 or 1998 I was going to Mankato State University. I was a black belt in aikido, cross training in goju ryu karate and judo. I had just read *Autumn Lightning: The Education of an American Samurai,* by Dave Lowry.

In the book there is a story of a young samurai who seeks out training from a sword master. After the master finally accepts him as a student, he begins a series of grueling and unusual training methods. One of these methods is that the master would wait until the samurai was engrossed in one of the many menial, tedious tasks (cooking, cleaning, gathering firewood, daily life . . .) required of an apprentice, and then jump out and whack him with a bokken.

At first the samurai would get knocked out. Then he would barely get out of the way but spill all the food or firewood. Eventually the samurai would evade or block the bokken with the lid from the teapot or the kindling he was carrying, continuing on about his business. Only then would the master allow him to pick up a sword.

I decided that I needed to re-create that training experience for myself. At that time I was living at the fraternity house with twenty- to thirty-some odd guys.

I chose five guys that lived at the house, had classes with me, and knew my schedule. Basically they had access to me twenty-four hours a day. I gave these guys a big piece of neon-colored chalk (the kind kids use to write on driveways), roughly the size of a tanto.

I made a bet with them that if they could leave a chalk mark on me in a vital area (not just counting coup or point sparring), I would buy them dinner, and they could sign the clothing they marked and I would have to wear it for twenty-four hours, letting everyone know who "killed" the great and powerful Kasey. They got one chance for a lethal attack. I had one chance to block/ evade. I promised I wouldn't lock, throw, or strike them—just block/evade.

Some lessons that stuck with me:

- Awareness

- Reading terrain

- Improvised weapons

- Threat assessment

- Counter-ambush

- Midbrain or monkey brain—my kryptonite

- Violence dynamics

I didn't have terms to express the lessons I learned until I started reading and training with Marc [MacYoung] and Rory. Many professionals have experienced these concepts and realities for themselves. However, it is difficult to express in words and even more difficult to convey to others. Luckily Marc and Rory have been developing a common lexicon of terms to express the realities of violence. Like Syd Hoar's book *The A–Z of Judo*, where he lists all the different names the same technique goes by. When I read that book I was like, "I know that technique, only I call it X." With the realities of violence it's like, "I've experienced X, only I call it Y." I played this game in '97, but I will use terms I've recently adopted into my teaching method to convey the lessons I learned.

As Paul Harvey used to say, here is the rest of the story.

Just playing the game improved my awareness. Again, becoming actively aware that you are looking for anomalies in pattern makes a tremendous difference in the identification and assessment.

First I was looking for those five guys, which was fairly easy. Then those guys would give the chalk to other guys I didn't know were playing the game. However, unless you're a sociopath hunting and killing people, even just playing at hunting and killing people is hard. There are telltale signs. Subconscious weapons checks, hiding hands, target glances.

They came at me when I was sleeping, they came at me when I was eating, they came at me at school, and I was very successful at detecting and deflecting their attacks. How was I killed, you ask? A lot of these attack-prevention skills are used by your forebrain. I was killed when I was forced into my midbrain or "monkey brain."

Monkey brain is where the term "monkey dance" comes from. Basically your monkey brain is concerned with the Fs: fight, flight, freeze, feed, and fornicate. I used "fornicate" because my dad says I use *fuck* too much in my writing. I hear you thinking, "Kasey, you didn't answer the question. How did you get killed?"

OK, so my buddy who is beautifully devious was dating a very attractive girl. She reminded me of Neve Campbell, and she had a belly ring (this is back when belly rings were new and exotic and only for women who had nice tummies). So he gives her the chalk. She blatantly flirts and uses her feminine wiles. All my samurai skills of awareness and threat assessment (forebrain) turn off. Monkey brain takes over. All the monkey can handle is fight, flight, freeze, feed, and fornicate. So where my forebrain should have thought:

- I have a girlfriend.
- She has a boyfriend (my good buddy).
- Why is she acting like this?
- Basically looking for anomalies in pattern.

My monkey brain thought:

- Boobies.
- Tummy.
- She totally digs me.
- Ouch. How did I get stabbed with chalk?

Good thing I had an understanding girlfriend (she eventually married me).

The "temptress" used social skills to commit asocial violence. That's how I got killed.

And now you know the rest of the story.

So how can I prevent getting killed in this manner? Learn how to prevent or delay the monkey brain from taking over.

Kasey described not only how a global awareness drill is set up, but was able to analyze his vulnerabilities after the fact. "Stupid things

I do that can get me killed" are things you want to find out in training, not in real life.

Do this: design a global awareness exercise incorporating these considerations:

- Real risk. The cost of losing could be pain, embarrassment of singing in public, wearing a shirt with the winner's name, or buying a dinner on a student's budget, but it has to hurt to lose.

- Incomplete control. You don't get to know all the rules. Kasey's friends recruited others. He didn't see that coming the first time.

- Train for what you are training for. The purpose of a global awareness drill is to detect danger, not to practice impromptu knife fighting.

- As important as real danger might be, you have to make it safe on a number of levels:

  ○ You don't want people to get injured, so safe training weapons are actually better than unarmed attack. Part of what you need to sense is commitment.

  ○ You don't want anybody going to jail. This is simply covered by recruiting smart friends. Smart friends will recognize that they don't want to draw a scene or attract attention at something that, at a distance, might look like an attack or a fight. Excellent, because real criminals don't want witnesses either. This safety factor makes it more realistic, not less so.

- No safe times or safe places. You might want them or think you need them. You don't. If a place is safe, it should be because you made it safe, not because of an artificial rule that can become a habit of thought.

- Throughout the exercise and again afterward, you should have personal "debriefings" where you go over the lessons that you have learned in each encounter and each encounter avoided.

A lot of people have talked and written about the Cooper color codes. White for oblivious in a safe place, yellow for on alert, orange for imminent danger, red for under attack.

I have heard at least one instructor say you can't live in condition yellow. That's not true. Not only is condition yellow perfectly natural, it is not stressful or paranoid. It is *energizing*. It is simply paying attention. The same skill that will let you know when a human predator is disturbing the flow around you will let you know that the gulls are swarming a school of fish you can't see, or read tracks in the frost or smell a change in the weather. There is nothing special about condition yellow. It is just living, aware, in the moment. It is natural for all animals.

Any time you spend in condition white, you aren't living anyway.

Legal Articulation

WV

Most of the readers will not have a grounding in force law. If you do, this exercise is simple.

Do this: choose a news article about self-defense or an officer using force. From that article, derive the elements of a self-defense claim and articulate why or why not the force used was legal. Do this every time you read such an article, especially if the article is trying to be sensationalistic.

The elements justifying force can be divided into three "threat factors":

Did the threat have the intent to harm? Intent is not always conscious. Someone running over you because of texting while driving is just as much of a threat as someone who deliberately set out to kill you by automobile. Lenny in *Of Mice and Men* killed things he thought he was only petting. Don't confuse this with legal culpability of the threat. You are justifying the necessity of your defense, not what the attacker could be charged with.

Did the threat have the means to cause harm? "Means" is simply ability. A knife or gun is obvious means for a lethal threat. But so are size and fists or boots. Was the threat capable of harm and, if so, of how much harm?

Did the threat have the opportunity to cause harm? In other words, could the threat reach the intended victim with the means?

Examples may make things a little clearer. If you have ever seen a two-year-old in a tantrum, you have seen pure, murderous intent. Completely without conscience, the child would kill or destroy anything he could. Godzilla destroying Tokyo could not match a two-year-old for vicious *intent*.

However, a two-year-old lacks the means to be a credible threat. He simply isn't big or strong enough to carry out his intentions.

A man with a knife is a lethal threat. He has the means. However, if he can't reach you (you are locked in your house or car, or he is far away), he lacks opportunity.

All three must be present: intent, means, and opportunity, *or* the threat must be intent on developing a lacking element. Jack Nicholson's character in *The Shining* had murderous *intent* and a fire ax for *means*. If he were breaking down your door to create *opportunity*, you would not need to wait for him to get all the way in before you cap his ass.

For civilian self-defense, there is often a fourth element: preclusion (in most states. Always check your local laws). In order for it to be self-defense, you must show that there was no other option. There was no opportunity to run or talk, or those options would not have worked.

Preclusion does not apply to peace officers. Cops have a duty to act. They are usually forbidden, by policy or statute, from running away from dangerous situations.

The intent, means, and opportunity make for a threat of a specific level . . . and the level of the threat authorizes a certain amount of force.

The bottom line is this: *for a claim of self-defense, one must use the minimum level of force that one reasonably believes is necessary to safely resolve the situation.*

Officers are held to a similar standard.

Minimum level of force means the following:

- If presence is enough (witnesses tend to make bad guys quit being bad), you don't use more.
- If verbal force is enough (ranging from reasoning to screaming to getting help), you don't use more.
- If touch is enough (push, pull, hold, takedown), you don't use more.
- If pain is enough, you don't use more.
- If damage is enough, you don't use more.
- Only if nothing else is enough do you use lethal force.

There is also the doctrine of competing harms. Lethal force is only authorized if imminent death or serious injury is threatened. In most jurisdictions, lasting harm (damage) is inappropriate in defending property.

Reasonably believe means that you cannot be held responsible for things that you could not have known. If you saw a 280-pound man swinging a club at you, that is what you knew. When it comes out that the threat was a child of fifteen, that cannot be used against you. It also means you will not be expected to make a decision in a half-second that some self-proclaimed expert came to after days of deliberation. Further, there is a lot of case law trying to define "reasonable." In real life, it means when the jury hears your story, they would have done about what you did.

It also means that fear alone does not justify force. It must be a reasonable fear. If you have been terrified of clowns since you were a child, that fear does not magically turn your clown-murdering spree into self-defense.

Necessary is the word that necessitates preclusion.

Safely is a reminder that self-defense is not a contest or a game. You are not required to give the bad guy a fair chance. You use enough force to get out in one piece. If a citizen or an officer is trying to save another person and takes extra risk to do it, not only does he fail to save the victim, but he also becomes a part of the problem. Resources (other officers or paramedics or involved bystanders) who might have been available to save the victims are wasted trying to save the "hero." If you want to help others, you have a responsibility to stay in one piece.

Resolve means simply to end it. If you lock onto one solution and miss an easier, more obvious way, you have failed at preclusion. Running away resolves most self-defense situations as effectively as fighting, and without force. More effectively, in most instances.

The situation must be *yours*. If you create the situation or decide something is your job that is not (like making the guys in the back of the theater be quiet), you might use force, but it is unlikely you'll be able to claim self-defense. The patrons of a club cannot throw out obnoxious people. The owner, manager, or the owner's designee (the bouncers) may. Officers, if they are called, may or must.

Remember that in any use of force, it is not an "average" situation. The force used to stop one threat will be insufficient to stop several. Weapons, even weapons not in hand (e.g., standing next to a rack of kitchen knives), may require more, faster force than an unarmed threat. If there is no opportunity to escape and no guarantee of how much force the threat will use if he renders the victim helpless, the victim must use any force available to prevent becoming helpless.

When the victim is surprised, there is no time or information to finely grade an appropriate amount of force. The victim must use as much force as is available to get safe enough to make those distinctions.

A younger, stronger, bigger threat will require more force than an elderly, unhealthy, smaller threat.

A threat in an altered state of consciousness may not only be incapable of understanding speech, but may not respond to pain or any lower level of force, and may even ignore damage.

Look at the circumstances and the different comparative factors between the people involved.

And so, the exercise is simple.

Do this: when you read a news story about a force situation, articulate your reasoning. Was the force necessary? Was there a threat with intent, means, and opportunity? Were there other options (preclusion)? Identify the specific force used as a level. Was there a lower level that would have worked safely and reliably? Why or why not?

Then, most important of all, explain as you would to a jury why this level of force was appropriate. Do not try to explain why it wasn't appropriate. If you ever use force, you will likely make a life-altering decision in a fraction of a second. It will not be cognitive or planned or reasoned. It will be based on good, if subconscious, decisions. Assume, for the purpose of this exercise, that you made the exact decision the person in the article made and explain it.

World Building

This is a thought experiment for a group. I'm occasionally asked to give classes on realistic violence for writers. Sometimes the disconnects are pretty deep. People have been very conditioned by the films they have watched and the stories they have read to expect violence to happen in a certain way. Often the physicality of it is wrong: short people don't and can't fight like tall people, arms only reach so far, a sword has so much momentum, and you can't just reverse the stroke with a flick of your wrist . . .

But often, everything is wrong. The fights happen for reasons that wouldn't be reasons to any real professionals. And the villains act like people with ego issues, not hunger or vengeance issues. And both act like they live in a world where loss has no more impact than watching your football team lose on television.

Do this: the world building exercise starts with choosing one of the basic survival modes of early humanity, whether the participants want to work from the viewpoint of a hunter-gatherer society or an early farming society. The people can discuss what those choices mean about the skills to get food and how children are raised and what are considered virtues and how deviance is handled . . . all from the baseline reminder that this is a world where people starve.

Then you introduce the "to save my children" (TSMC) exercise (IW7):

If no one were going to help you and there were a very real possibility your children would starve tomorrow, what would you be willing to do? Steal, rob, murder, prostitute yourself, prostitute your children . . . ?

The TSMC exercise uses the paradigm to understand a certain type of modern criminal. In world building, it is followed up differently:

This has been the baseline for most people for most of human history.

The exercise works as a group discussion at first. What strategies would work to safely kill strangers for food or money? Who would you target? Would you prey on people in your own community? Or would that weaken the tribe too much?

And how would you make the kill?

As much as possible, the students work through this. They will benefit from some guidance from someone who has thought about it deeply. For instance, consider that preying on insiders would decrease resources. That equates very well with the fact that betrayal triggers the most extreme levels of violence in the real world.

For writers, I then ask if their antagonists are attacking in ways that are congruent with their motivations. In self-defense circles I have them compare the attacks they designed with the defenses they train.

We then discuss basic strategy, and I suggest two: raiders and lurers. Raiders will go out and take things from other tribes. The lurers will entice people to come to them. One example of luring that everyone recognizes after a few seconds of thought is the story of Hansel and Gretel. In a world where children are abandoned to starve so there will be enough food for the parents, what better lure for a cannibal than a house seemingly made of gingerbread?

The group then divides, one to create a raider society, the other to create a lurer society.

Then the questions:

1. If you are willing to murder for food or money, what story do you tell yourself? We are humans, and no matter what we do, we will convince ourselves that we are the good guys. What mechanism do you use to justify premeditated and socially sanctioned murder?

   Note well: I'm fairly cool with "Because I don't want my children to die." But very few people are cool with simple justifications on big issues. They want something greater.

2. What story do you tell your children?

3. How do you teach them to kill, both the mechanics of it and the justifications? Seriously, how do you explain to a six-year-old why it is OK to kill a Taboolian but not OK to hit his sister?

4. Would the societies exploit without killing? Can the raiders demand tribute instead of killing and taking? Would they take slaves or would slaves slow them down? The lurers killing people for food

or money—would they ever consider taking one with special skills alive? Would that be too great a security risk? How much would it change society?

5. Social controls. Raiders require teamwork, discipline, and clear lines of authority to survive. Lurers will either starve or be massacred if word gets out about what they do. What do you do with tribesmen who aren't trustworthy?

6. Lesser levels of social control: How are disputes handled within a tribe that is very good at killing? Remember that killing tribe members weakens you in battle with others. In class after class, this question is the one that gets the students thinking about ritualized fighting—duels to first blood, nonlethal unarmed combat, stylized sport fighting. Martial arts, in other words.

7. What happens when the tribe is no longer hungry? It will be generations after the original stories were invented. If the tribal gods demanded sacrifice (really to justify gathering food or wealth), will they continue to demand the same? Even when food and wealth are plentiful? What will the people in charge of the stories do to remain in power? How long will it take and what influences for a cultural identity story to change?

8. If the group is threatened by another group of outsiders, how does the group imagine, plan, and thus conduct war? It will be less a problem for a raider society, where sacking and pillaging are just part of being a man, but for an overtly peaceful society like many lurers . . . how do you get people to fight, teach them to fight? Do you create a new myth or get a new prophecy? Hire mercenaries? Try to adapt the luring tactics to war and poison a peace delegation?

9. If you do go to war and one member of the tribe is very, very good at killing people and seems to enjoy it, what do you do with him during peacetime? He is a hero in wartime, someone people fear at least a bit in peacetime. Do you need extra controls on the proven warriors? If so, what? And who enforces that level of control?

On one level or another, all of these problems still exist.

World building is a thought and discussion experiment, but people have unwittingly re-created historical societies from the Thuggee to the Mongols playing it, sometimes in eerie detail.

For analysis:

Do you see parallels between the types and strategies of modern criminals? Do many violent criminals have a personal mythology?

Do we as humans assume that the mythology came first and the behavior followed? When we do make that assumption, we kind of forget there was a need underlying it all.

This will likely offend some people, but try to give it some honest thought: how many religions suddenly make more sense when you start looking at them as justifying lies for children? How many of the purposes behind the myths simply no longer apply? Right and wrong may or may not change over time, but resources to fulfill needs do, and that drives a lot of the rules.

Personal Threat Assessment   WW1

There are a very limited number of types of interpersonal violence, and each of those follows a specific logic. Each has predictable goals and parameters. The implication, of course, is that each person is more vulnerable to certain types of bad stuff than other types of bad stuff.

To go into this exercise in depth requires some background. For more information, read the section on violence dynamics in *Facing Violence*.

Very quickly: Social violence, and the more common social conflict, center on aspects of group identity and tend to be less dangerous. The specific triggers are usually as follows:

- Group membership. Some groups have initiation rights with violence. Some groups draw lines with some level of what might be called violence. Gang colors are protected, possibly with more force, but with the same dynamic as fans feel about their sports teams.

- Territory protection. Many groups, if not most, will discourage outsiders. How violent that will be is cultural. A stranger walking into a redneck watering hole will be treated differently than the same stranger walking into a private yacht club or the grounds of a Colombian drug lord.

- Territory access. There are places generally considered open to the public, like certain bars, where newcomers will be given a challenge.

- Determining the hierarchy. Probably the most common—straight-up dominance fistfights.

- Enforcing the rules. All groups have rules. In functional groups that disapprove of violence, a glance or a quick word is all the enforcement necessary. In different groups, rules may be enforced with anything from a letter of reprimand to a beating or an execution. The most extreme levels of violence are reserved for people who have betrayed their own group.

Asocial violence is directed outside the tribe. It is more similar to hunting or slaughtering than fighting. These are the basic types:

- Resource predation—crime, violent or not, committed for money. Drug addiction requires a lot of cash and drives a lot of crime, both violent and nonviolent.

- Process predation—the rarest type. There are certain people who enjoy hurting other people, including rape and murder. Some will say that committing their crime of choice is the only time they feel alive.

There are a handful of places where violence is likely to happen:

- Where young men gather in groups.

- Where people get their minds altered. (Combine those two and you have bars.)

- Where territories, real or imagined, are in dispute. (Combine all three and you have the potential for soccer riots.)

- Where you don't know the rules.

- And, last, predatory violence tends to happen in lonely places.

A personal threat profile is taking this information, as well as anything you know from other sources or learned from exercises IW8 or WW4 and WW5, and applying that information to you.

If you are a young, strong, fit martial athlete, are you a likely target for a mugging (resource predator)? Would you be on the list of preferred victims? Probably not . . . unless you already have some bad habits, such as flashing rolls of cash in strip clubs to try to impress people.

On the other hand, big healthy guys get monkey-dance challenges more. The math is better. If the person wins or you back down, that's a lot of status. Even if the person loses, they get points for "heart," trying someone bigger.

Do this: complete your personal threat profile. Then do some profiles for other people. You'll find some disturbing truths about the way the world works. The strong young men who train for violence are only targets for the safest and most predictable types—the social violence.

The untrained, the small, and the weak are the targets for predation. Those least likely to develop the skills are the ones most likely to need them, and the guy who looks the toughest will consistently be the least tested . . . except for situations he contributes to.

SC: SPARRING AND COMPETITION

You haven't seen a lot of competitive drills in here. That's because of my bias. Intense competition teaches very valuable lessons, things you *cannot* learn in any other way, but they are different than the things you learn in other drills.

Most of my student base is more than competitive enough. They know how to dig deep, they try to stay in better condition . . . but that isn't always conducive to learning efficiency.

Someone who decides to act competitively in a cooperative drill will seem to do really well, just like the guy who pulls a gun in a chess match. And he'll learn about as much.

I encourage competition, but you need to keep a very clear head. Almost everything that makes unarmed martial arts competition possible, at any level of intensity, is a bad survival habit. Yet because the experience is so intense, the lessons of competition seem "more truer" and the habits ingrain harder.

What will sparring do for you?

It really depends. Noncontact striking *kumite* (punches and kicks) may teach you a bit about strategy and may teach you many neat but overly complicated lessons about timing. It will also train you to miss, especially at speed and under stress. It will ruin your distancing. If you are good at point sparring, it will give you an entirely unjustified sense of confidence.

Judo or grappling of any type will teach you how to really move a body that doesn't want to be moved, and that is a valuable skill. I've learned far more about applied structure from judo coaches than any "internal artist" so far. You will learn to take impact in a throwing art to a great level and go beyond fears of losing balance and falling. You'll also get very hard to knock down.

You'll get used to the close-contact feel of a sweating, struggling body.

On the other hand, you will be trained away from finishing things quickly or escaping. You will be imprinting a need to dominate, which is an entirely different thing than the skill to prevail.

If you do hard contact or full contact, you will learn that you can take a punch and how to take one and how to recover. You will learn better than anywhere else how to put kinetic energy into a moving body. You will learn about pain. In many ways, the essence of survival fighting is the ability to move through damage to deliver damage. Without experiencing full-contact hits, the very nature of fighting will be a mystery to you, no matter how hard you train in other aspects.

The biggest danger in sparring comes from intensity. It feels more real. Bad information received intensely will affect you more deeply than good information with less intensity. In the section that follows I won't go into how to set up matches or play. Instead, I will concentrate on what I consider to be the valuable lessons and the dangers.

Kumite and Variations

By kumite I mean point sparring. A noncontact game of strategy and speed.

In many ways, kumite is a collection of bad training that feels good. Two people, head to head, using similar techniques, going for complete domination through technique and all done without (much) pain or injury. Sounds good, huh?

But pain and injury are the natural elements of the fight. To train without those is to learn to swim without water.

Pulling your strikes, no matter how much it demonstrates "control," is practicing to miss. Thousands and thousands of reps teaching your body and hindbrain, creating neural pathways to "win" by missing.

It screws up distancing—"just out of reach" becomes the right range for a technique, and that is not only out of range to touch, but penetrating damage requires you to get even closer. All of your defenses work better with just a little more distance, a little more time ... and so defenses that fail in an assault become common in point sparring.

Kumite is sometimes touted as a place to learn strategy and timing. There is an element to that, but it is dueling strategy, the strategy of feints and counters, that works when you see something coming and have agreed to meet at a specified place and time.

For a long time, I thought the value in it was just the fun. I enjoyed it and I enjoy speed games. Kumite was, to my mind, a lot like table tennis: fun, but not really applicable to fighting.

But there is a skill there, if you play right. It is a variation on the maai with weapons drill (F1). Kumite can teach you to read a body.

There are positions and a distance where a threat can hit you with no telegraph. For the most part, you try to prevent someone from getting this advantage in kumite, but kumite can teach you to recognize it. And that's good, because an experienced bad guy will do everything in his power to get to this position before you have any idea an attack is coming.

It's rare, though. Most positions require at minimum a shift in the center of gravity before the person can hit with power. You learn to read that as well.

More commonly, there must be a shift as well as a change in foot position. Just as in sparring, we start out of range, and in order to attack us, a person has to get close. How someone will cross that distance and what attacks can be launched when he does are things you can learn to read.

If someone arouses your suspicions (if he doesn't, you're vulnerable), you can tell not only if he can attack, but what he would have to do in order to attack. You can predict aggressive actions.

Value: You learn to read physical possibility. Once you can do this, you can stay relaxed just beyond the critical distance.

Danger: It can mess you up concerning every aspect of a real fight, from distancing to timing to power generation to the natural environment.

Judo Randori: Nage

Every instructor has prejudices, and I love judo. So take everything I am about to say with the appropriate amount of salt. *Nage waza* randori is sparring aimed at throws. It will usually continue on the ground, but for my take on that, see SC3: "Free Grappling and Variations."

There's a lot missing in judo. You aren't allowed to strike in competition or put hands on the face, and those really make it easier to throw when you do it, and much harder to get close when the bad guy does it. But I don't see a lot of bad habits in judo.

You get used to moving a body. If you have an old-school instructor who thinks weight classes are an abomination, you will get extraordinary training in how to use momentum, and that is a key skill in handling bigger threats.

You get used to fighting at bad-breath range, and weird smells and sweaty bodies. And you get used to slamming into the ground again and again. It gets most people over their natural fear of impact.

There are a few problems with judo randori training. One is all of the chaos that is missing. I encourage judoka looking into self-defense to get their judo down and then go look for a good jujutsu instructor who can dirty it up.

I'm a jujutsu partisan. I love it, but I also recognize the weakness. Proper jujutsu is a very broad-based martial art. It not only includes locking, throwing, grappling, striking, strangling, and gouging, but it blends them and uses the mix to augment each element. Cool, huh?

And that's the weakness. Jujutsu is so broad based and there are so many ways to "cheat" that very, very few jujutsuka develop really clean technique. I joke sometimes that judo, aikido, and kenpo each took a third of the jujutsu curriculum and polished it until they felt safe.

If you are a jujutsuka, I encourage you to spend some serious time with pure strikers, pure grapplers—anyone who can help you perfect your skills.

Another is that the skills required turn judo into a chess game of balance. Which isn't necessarily a weakness unless you get addicted to the complexity. Throws, counterthrows, and setups are necessary to do well in judo. The other guy is playing the same game by the same rules, and often the trickier or more patient wins. Tricky and patient aren't nearly as useful under assault.

But, and this is sort of an advantage, judo techniques are easier to pull off in real life than they are in judo tournaments. A full-entry hip throw in judo requires exquisite timing and usually a way to distract your opponent or trick him into supplying half of the position. That's hard. I've heard one self-defense instructor say he didn't teach hip throws "because it is *never* a good idea to turn your back on an enemy." Which sounds sensible.

The thing is, in real life, people try to jump on your back. They hand you the hard part of the chess match. If you're ready for it.

Value: You learn how to move a body, one of the absolute fundamentals of dealing with violence.

Danger: Not much.

Free Grappling and Variations SC3

There are lots of rules for grappling and wrestling—gi or no gi; wrestling, judo, sambo, or Brazilian jiu-jitsu; with or without strikes; with or without different types of locks . . .

Here's the good: grappling is the premier way to learn to move a body, and moving a body, as previously mentioned, is one of the absolute fundamentals. I won't go so far as to say if you can't grapple, you can't fight, but it is damn close.

Do all fights go to the ground? No. But here's the deal. You don't get to pick where fights go. None of this unarmed stuff is for the best-case scenario. We train for the bad stuff. There's a reason it's called "self-defense" and not "turkey dinner at Grandma's."

But grappling is perfectly positioned to ingrain an ungodly number of bad habits.

It is fun.

It is almost exactly the way kids (and puppies and other small animals) play dominance games. It hits us at a very deep mental level.

Of all the arts out there, grappling is the one you can go hardest at with the lowest incidents of injury.

Those all seem like good things and they are, for *grappling*. Less so for surviving an attack.

It is fun. So some people will ignore less-fun training to play. Fun things tend to get dragged out. Can we agree that in the real world, with obstacles and bricks, broken bottles and sharp stuff, and threats who may not be working alone, staying on the ground is a bad idea? If so, the goal to submit instead of to get up ingrains a habit to stay and play longer than necessary. And I'm guilty of it myself. I was a judoka for a long time, loved it, and particularly loved groundwork . . . and every time an inmate and I hit the floor, I had to consciously fight the urge to go into tournament-judo mode, because I was good at it and I liked it.

Dominance games. One of the biggest issues with self-defense is that so many people have experience with social violence and try to deal with a predator the way they would deal with an angry family member or a friend getting cocky. Predators don't play the same game, and a little bit of cheating goes a long way.

An example, just to get you thinking: If you are a grappler, imagine a typical match at training. If your opponent had a knife, would you do things differently? If so, I submit that, for self-defense, when he didn't have a knife, you were doing it wrong. You were in the wrong mind-set for self-defense. Most practitioners grapple in the mind-set of a puppy playing at dominance.

You can go hard. Grappling is so perfectly suited for noninjurious dominance contests that every society in history had a grappling system. It is the perfect thing to teach young men so they can blow off steam safely.

And you go hard in the exact skills where it is safe to do so. It's not safe to strike throats or spines, so even when they are allowed, finishing strikes are pulled. So the match never ends with strikes, always with submissions. Your brain conditions to believe submissions are the only real goal . . .

Remember, before anyone gets upset—that's not a list of what is wrong with grappling. That is a list of why grappling habits ingrain so hard. It matches a lot of our human wiring. Which means bad habits will stick, as described above. But so will good habits.

Grappling is a premier self-defense skill, but in real application, under assault, grappling must serve a goal. Always. If your goal is to get away, submissions are incompatible with that goal. If your goal is to handcuff, none of the face-up pins apply. You grapple in order to do something else. You do not grapple to grapple.

Value: Premier training for moving a body.

Danger: Direct route to deep-brain conditioning. Be careful of what you condition.

Jujutsu Randori

Jujutsu randori was one of the drills my Sosuishitsu-ryu instructor, Dave Sumner, inflicted on us. Two people would start touching—chest touching chest, chest to flank, or chest to back. At the start signal it would be a no-holds-barred match. Beginners would start at half speed (no one could stay slow, though), and seniors would go full speed. For seniors, stiff contact except to the upper spine. Controlled contact for everyone.

I thought for years that this was the best fight simulation ever. No scripting, almost no rules, all targets in play, no techniques disallowed, standing or on the ground, sometimes with weapons or improvised weapons. And it is a blast.

It can be physically exhausting and dangerous. If you haven't done something like this, I would suggest a slow buildup. There is enough potential for damage that trust and control are required.

I'd been at it for decades before I found out the real value. It is good for brawling, but it does something else unique.

Many of the people Dave trained were superbly integrated fighters. I believe that came from this drill.

By starting very close, all of your techniques are in play. You can throw, lock, strike, gouge, strangle, bite . . . It is so fast and so close that you have to give up on using your eyes and fight by touch, which is faster than sight anyway. Offense and defense become a holistic unit and you learn to fight as "three." You do what you do and you control what the opponent does, and this four-legged creature with four arms and two heads and one shared center of gravity, well, you learn to run that too.

Value: Integrates all of your skills into a single thought.

Danger: Misses some of the context of an assault. And sometimes it's not safe.

Full Contact

SC

I think of boxing here, but muay Thai or Kyoshinkan karate fit just as well. Any sport where you will get hit and hit as hard as you can.

A detail first: Beware of your safety equipment. If you can do a technique in safety equipment that you can't safely do without it, you are conditioning a bad habit. To be specific, closed-fist punches to the face are a bad idea. I know people who swear by them, but I have sent at least nine deputies (and I do not know how many inmates) to the hospital after they broke their hands punching someone in the head with closed fists. Two of those have permanent injuries. One of those was a trained competitive amateur boxer.

I have never once sent someone to the hospital after receiving a single closed-fist punch to the head. Any technique that is more likely to cripple you than it is to incapacitate the bad guy is a *bad technique*.

That said, I firmly believe everyone should box. No one should stay with it for very long (microconcussions are not good for you), but everyone interested in self-defense should try it. Getting hit is the natural environment of a fight. You need to know what it feels like, and you need to learn that you can keep fighting. And if you can't keep fighting after getting hit, you need to stick with boxing until you can.

There are lots of little but important things you will learn under a good instructor in full contact that you won't learn anyplace else: how to hit hard while moving; how to hit a moving target; how to protect yourself and minimize the damage of incoming strikes; how to get an opponent into your strike zone; how to crash with total body commitment . . .

Lots of stuff. But the biggest thing that full-contact fighters tend to have that noncontact fighters miss is courage. And that's pretty damn important.

Value: Courage.

Danger: Long-term brain damage.

Mixed Martial Arts   SC6

MMA has become its own modern sport, but for our purposes, I'm including any competition style that has a full-contact striking component and a grappling component.

MMA has a lot of advantages of SC3: "Free Grappling" and SC5: "Full Contact." I believe there has been a long evolution to find the most extreme but relatively safe test of manhood possible. MMA is the current level of that evolution. You will get hit and hurt and you will be exhausted, and in the end, one person will have won and the other will have given up or been defeated.

So on top of learning to move a body and fighting to the goal and courage and skills, MMA adds one critical thing to the mix. By allowing a broader range of skills than boxing, muay Thai, wrestling, or judo, it allows the practitioners greater freedom in creating strategy. It is a thinking man's game, and I mean that in the very old-school sense of the word *man*.

Is there a problem? Absolutely, but it isn't in the competition. People mistake intensity for reality. If MMA competition is the most intense martial experience, it must be the most real, right?

If you are interested in dealing with violence, you have to understand this: everything is what it is, no more, no less, and no different. MMA may be the most intense competition, but a predator does everything he can to prevent his assault ever turning into a competition.

The essence of a contest is to show up at a given time in a given place to test your skills against someone in your own weight class who will use the same skills, and in the end everyone will know who was the best on that particular day.

Not a single thing in that description has any bearing on sudden violence. But, somehow, it has come to be called reality fighting.

Value: Probably the best thing ever designed to measure yourself as a man.

Danger: Don't get caught up believing it is other than that.

Competition

Up to now we've been talking about sparring, friendly in-house stuff with people you know. Competition is just sparring with strangers on one level. Not that different. But sometimes it seems that way.

Crowds and judges make a difference. Many people get more anxiety at the thought of being watched by a crowd than by the thought of being injured. The judges get to decide if what you did was good or not, no matter what happened or what they couldn't see.

You will see that even people who train in the same system as you fight differently. Some cheat, and some may feel that what you do is cheating. You will probably see the power of politics in martial arts up close and personal.

It is all artificial. The crowd, the lights, the referee. Everything except what you are doing: tying up and going for the throw or hitting and being hit.

I suggest that everyone try competition. Especially if you hate it. For that matter, any aspect of your training that you hate, you should make yourself do, because fighting is pretty damned unpleasant as well and doing unpleasant things should be a habit.

The adrenaline of being judged is somewhat closer to the adrenaline of being attacked than anything I get in sparring. It may be different for you.

The one critical thing about competition: You can't pretend you are good. Without this piece, anyone can print out a certificate or sew some stripes on a black belt, and people will listen and maybe be conned. That's also one of the things I love about judo: no matter who you are, you are going to get on the mat, and we will all know if you live up to your talk.

Value: Put up or shut up.

Danger: That some will forget it is entirely artificial.

INTERLUDE #5:
THE VIOLENCE-PRONE
PLAY GROUP

No matter how good your instructor is, if he or she can answer all of your questions, it means one of two things. Either you are very, very new or you are not thinking for yourself.

Just as I have biases and assumptions about violence and what we are training for, I have very deep beliefs about how we should train and why we train. At its very heart, I think any martial art or self-defense training is, or should be, about making each and every student stronger and more complete. Smarter, tougher, more aware. Also more independent. Which means that any training fostering dependency or hierarchies is actively sabotaging the student—provided survival and personal growth are the goals. If you are trying to re-create a culture that doesn't have the word *freedom* in its language and enforce a caste system, then that's a different thing.

At some point in your training, if you are training to be the best you can, you must get to a place where you are asking questions your instructors can't answer. If you don't, you will stagnate. For that matter, if you are the senior person in your region, you have to come up with a way to keep asking questions and finding answers or you will stagnate.

Our solution is the VPPG, or Violence-Prone Play Group. The members are all senior practitioners in their arts of choice. Most had become dissatisfied. Though they love their arts, you simply can't find all of your answers in the same bottle.

Selecting Members

This can be a big deal or not. We don't allow beginners because we aren't there to teach. Sometimes we are all a little sick of teaching and want to get back in learning mode. That said, everyone is a beginner at something (most things in a vast world), so even that isn't a hard-and-fast rule. I could see a group of beginners making headway with this model.

What is necessary is trust. Sometimes we play at the edges of what is safe. I'll do things with my VPPG that I wouldn't consider, for liability and safety reasons, doing with a class or a private student. I have to trust each and every member's control (both physical skill and emotional/ego) and honesty. We are getting together to see what works, which means no going along or helping a technique or trying to look good.

None of the members is shy. That's not strictly true. Two of us are. But we aren't shy in the group. If you keep insight to yourself, it is wasted. Communication without information is noise, but information without communication is waste. Everyone in the group has to be assertive enough to share.

Last, the VPPG should have the widest mix of backgrounds you can find. You don't want the group to be too big. Getting one senior practitioner from the military, civilian, and police arts of each country with a martial tradition would run into the hundreds. That said, different training backgrounds see problems in entirely different ways. The more ways you can see a problem, the more options you have to deal with it.

Our hard core of three includes a modern/eclectic/boxing/competition history, Indonesian/weapon/shadowy past, and classical Japanese jujutsu/competitive judo/LEO defensive tactics. The ones who show up when they can range from modern jujitsu to hapkido, to the old silverback who has studied everything, pure DTs, and MMA. (I don't have a really good senior traditional Chinese guy available on this coast.)

Structure of a Meeting

The VPPG runs like this: one person throws out his "mystery." Frequently, with our group, it centers more on how to teach than how to do, but not always. Then all the members brainstorm solutions. Then we go bang it out and see what works.

New Guy (NG) goes first. He's a classically trained martial artist: I'm not happy with our gun disarms.

Cop Background (CB): Take a step back on that. It's not just a physical thing. When and how is it going to come up? The most common I see are at convenience stores, and I don't see anybody teaching disarms with a store counter between you and the threat. If someone is just threatening you for money, you give up the money.

NG: What if he was going to kill you anyway?

CB: Then the question becomes, Why hasn't he already? It's a narrow window, not of time but of, I dunno, circumstance, where it matters. Someone who doesn't want to kill you but is in reach and a situation that justifies taking that kind of risk.

Women's Self-Defense Background (WSD): Intimidating a victim to a secondary crime scene.

Everyone agrees that this is both the most likely and most realistic problem. Next, how is the situation going to develop? Probability of approach in a public or semipublic area versus an isolated area?

WSD: Public or semipublic. Someone approaching in an isolated area triggers different responses earlier, and if it's a blitz attack, the disarm scenario doesn't come into play.

Approach? We play with a bunch of different ones. Hair and collar grip draw too much attention. Insufficient control with wrist. Upper arm grip with off hand (or around the shoulders) and handgun against threat's belly pointed at victim's liver.

Silat Background (SB): Try turning into him, using the gun as the pivot point.

CB: It's going to pan her arm.

Old Guy Who's Done Everything (OG): It's going to pan his hand too, but I don't think his reaction speed will be fast enough. Who brought the Airsoft?

No one did. We'll play live later.

WSD (the smallest) works the technique on SB (the biggest).

NG: Body mechanics are OK, but what now? Arm lock?

CB: No way. Arm is bent. She'd need to be much stronger to have a chance at pulling off an armbar.

OG: And he has a free hand, and size.

SB: I like the brainstem shot.

CB: But you're tall, have arms like an orangutan and great structure. [WSD] couldn't even reach that target.

SB: She needs a shutdown though.

CB: What about trailing knee, sprinting through his knee?

OG: Or stomping on the knee?

NG: I'm still uncomfortable with her giving up control of the gun.

SB: He's bigger and stronger. If she attempts to stay in control, it's going to turn into a wrestling match and she'll lose. What she needs is an exit strategy. We're just trying to come up with the safest possible way.

CB: Ear slap? She can reach it. It's not protected by the shoulder like your brainstem shot. And it's the only strike I've never seen fail. Have any of you seen it fail?

Long talk ensues about definitions of failure, number of times members have used, received, or seen percussive ear slaps and whether they really caused concussions or it just so happens that a ruptured eardrum mimics a severe concussion . . .

Practice. Play. Test to failure. Other options. Consensus: It's not a 100 percent option, but nothing in real life is.

Then . . .

OK, [SB], you're up. What are you working on?

SB: I've been trying to figure out how to teach . . .

T: TRICKS AND ONE-OFFS

These aren't actually drills. They are exercises that you demonstrate once to show a deeper truth. Most will not work on the same person a second time. Some will learn to game it.

Most of my favorites I will not describe here. Not just to tease you. One of the things about tricks is that when you read about them, you think you understand, and you may not fall for that particular trick . . . but the underlying weakness is still there and you are still vulnerable.

Reread C5: "The Reception Line." In many ways, it is a one-off. It can be used for good continuing training, particularly in staying both relaxed and alert, in disguising readiness, how to identify armed people, and flipping the switch to counterassault mode. But much of the value for martial artists, the first time, is that they get a shattering insight into how many imaginary rules they bring to a situation and all the things they have learned not to see and not to think about.

As much as teaching gives new insights, sometimes it also applies blinders.

The Touchstone

T

You must first pick a demonstration partner. I prefer someone I don't know, who has excellent breakfall skills and preferably the best-known or most experienced martial artist available.

I take him in front of the class, turn so we are both facing the students shoulder to shoulder, and ask him to introduce himself to the class.

When he starts talking, I turn suddenly and fire a flurry of punches (noncontact) at his face, sweep his legs out from under him, and continue the flurry on the ground, stopping when he unfreezes and starts to react.

What is going on in the demo: This is how bad guys set up assaults. They get position first. Then they get the victim distracted. Then the threat attacks full out—no defense, no feinting or sparring. Even without contact it works reliably because it spikes the victim's OODA loop.

Each fist coming at the victim's face is an observation, a piece of information. If the victim can't orient, decide, and act before the next fist comes in (the new observation), the loop resets. In other words, unless you have conditioned yourself to act when overwhelmed, fast fists freeze you. Even when they don't hit.

The purpose of the demonstration is partially to show how bad guys attack. The setup, the explosiveness. It is largely to show that almost everything most martial artists have learned about timing and distancing was never intended for assault survival and doesn't work there. I call this the touchstone, and it is only a piece.

For surviving sudden violence, this is the touchstone—fast, unexpected, from the flank or behind. Overwhelming speed and damage. Designed to freeze your mind, hurt your body, and break your will. And there is still a piece missing from the demo. The bad guy is not going to pick the martial artist who moves best in the whole class. He's going to pick you when you are tired or injured. He will pick the old and the small.

"Hit Me as Hard as You Can"   T2

This one requires immense judgment. You need to be able to read people well. It will not work for you if you have a certain reputation. This is early-in-your-career stuff.

The demo is simple. You hand someone a club and tell him to hit you in the head as hard as he can. Then you do nothing. You do not move.

Most will wind up, swing, and when they see you not moving, do everything in their power to stop the strike. One of the people I used for this strained a muscle in his back stopping.

This is, obviously, not a safe demo. There are certain people who won't stop, but they are rarer than I think they should be. Antisocial personality disorders, people even mildly on the autism spectrum, and people with serious exposure to weapon violence will probably follow through.

Everyone will follow through if you have a reputation for having a lot of nifty moves. Hence, this is only something you can do with new students or early in your career.

This was one of the core aspects of my jujutsu kata training. We were expected to wait in stillness under a committed attack until the point where the uke could not shift or change. The primary purpose of that aspect of training, for us, was to be able to slow time and then move explosively. One of the side benefits is that you got very good at reading who would follow through and who would pull.

The purpose of the demo is what I call "glitch hunting." Everyone has some issues with using force on another human. Many people who think they are ready to hit a man in the head with a stick are not. This shows that.

In debriefing, the point to emphasize is that this was not a conscious decision to avoid hitting. This was all of your conditioning taking over in midswing. It can really screw you up when and if you need to take someone out.

The No-Touch Parry

This is a parlor trick. No more. It is something you do to demonstrate how much the mind can be influenced to control the body and how powerful communication is. Most fights are social violence and they are all about sending messages.

You need one physical skill: the ability to snap your fingers with either hand.

I demonstrate this on any given individual only once, but I am not sure that is necessary. And I avoid antisocial personality disorders, people on the autism spectrum, and those who have a history of dedicated, professional unarmed violence. If someone doesn't blink often, that is one of the clues to the first two.

Antisocials are wired to not care about people and thus miss a lot of the subconscious communication. People on the autism spectrum miss almost all subtle communication. Professionals (not all, but ideally) will make the decision and act despite cues.

Instruct the person to hit you in the chin. Preferably from long range with a karate lunge punch. (Clearly, this is not demonstrating a combat skill, understand?)

Using your mirror-side hand (your left hand if he is punching with his right, your right if he is punching with your left) at chest level, snap your fingers and point to the side. His fist will follow the point, and he will miss you.

This is not a combat skill or magic or useful in a real fight. The purpose is to show the students some of their own internal wiring. We are communicating animals. We follow instructions, sometimes even when it is not in our best interest. If a trained striker will miss when he is subtly instructed to, what are the odds that he will freeze if someone yells "*freeze!*"? How many grapplers will reflexively release pressure when the other guy taps, even if it isn't a game?

And some of those tricks, especially combining communication with your physical skills, can be useful.

Action/Reaction

This requires specialized equipment. With the sheriff's office we used Simguns (real firearms modified to fire subcaliber marking rounds) and armor. Anytime you use projectiles or weapons, take maximal safety precautions.

This drill was a valuable part of training rookies to understand how fast certain decisions must be made. Too many had been raised on television westerns and believed in the fastest draw.

I would act as the bad guy, with a loaded Simgun dangling at my side. Bric, my partner, would often demonstrate with his back turned and the gun held up like he was surrendering. Two officers, with loaded Simguns aimed at my center chest and fingers on the trigger, would order me to drop the weapon. Sometimes I would comply. When I didn't comply, I could reliably raise the gun and get at least two shots off before either officer could fire. If I sidestepped when I fired, both of the officers would miss, locked into aiming where I used to be.

The person who moves first almost always wins. It's the OODA loop. If the bad guy's act is your observe, he is three steps ahead of you in the process.

If you decide to give the guy the first move—unless he is slow, stupid, drunk, or telegraphs badly—you will eat the first hit.

There are things that can be tweaked in the drill to give lessons. First of all, both officers are giving commands. Switching from talking to fighting (unarmed or with weapons) seems to slow things down. Not talking, your reaction time is much better. The officers always stood shoulder to shoulder, though we never instructed them to. Had they spread out to triangulate me, the complexity would have increased and my speed would have been hampered. Could have shot one, but not both. Had the officers used cover, I would have had to think more and been slowed down.

Sometimes we would then reverse the drill, and I would play the officer. The student/bad guy expected the same pattern: weapons presented, verbal commands, and the bad guy makes the decision.

Instead, I would leap at him screaming, "Drop the weapon! Do it now!" and my weapon would be in his face and usually he would be down before he realized the pattern had changed.

Lessons here: Action beats reaction for good guys too. Interrupting an expected pattern slows people down (in OODA loop terms, it takes more time to orient). Verbal commands added to physical assault increase the freeze.

Interestingly, I've done a similar drill without a weapon of any kind, but making a motion of the draw while closing and screaming . . . and had both subjects and people watching from the class clearly see a gun that wasn't there.

T4 is a one-off because after a few officers had seen the demo, they'd just shoot me out of hand, and that wasn't the response we were trying to condition for the street.

Gush

The students had a pretty good idea what was coming. They knew I'd told them to bring their knives. They knew I had stopped by a butcher shop and gone to a thrift store for a bunch of old clothes. So they weren't surprised when I came out with bundles of something wrapped in T-shirts and hung them by strings in the training area.

Intellectually, everyone knows how dangerous a knife can be. Any decent weapon—hell, any decent kitchen knife—can go through clothing and muscle like it isn't even there. (If yours can't, you need to do some sharpening.)

So the group had a pretty good idea what to expect—a suspended slash and then a clinical look at how much cloth and meat the knife had severed.

Nope. The students who had flown me in for a few days of private lessons were also the students of one of the premier reality-based instructors in the States. I wanted to see how well their instructor had prepared them.

True, there was a nice cut of round steak rolled up inside several layers of rolled-up shirts. But inside each roll of steak was a can of warm shaken cherry cola.

Credit to the students and the instructor, some slashed, some thrust, but either way, the target exploded in a gush of warm, wet, sticky, nauseatingly sweet-smelling liquid, and none of them hesitated. They went to town. One pretty much destroyed her knife driving it into the meat again and again after it fell to the concrete. No hesitation. Good students of a good instructor.

It's my opinion that using a knife really isn't much of a technical skill. Maybe dueling would get really nuanced, but dueling knife on knife is high on the list of stupid ways to die. Darwin would approve. As the saying goes, there is one thing worse than coming in second in a knife fight, and that is tying for first.

Taking the dueling myth out of it, knives aren't used to win fights; knives are used to kill people—or in some cases, to intimidate. That's not what I'm talking about here. And that's not hard. Get the target unaware. Distract the target. Control the near arm or the head. Thrust to or near vascular or hollow organs. If you want to be really fancy, have your weapon hand make a circle before or as you pull the weapon out. Repeat as quickly as possible. Staccato thrusts.

Remember my bias—my concern was and is people who learned to shank in prison. Walk-by hamstringings were the attack of choice for a certain demographic not too long ago. If you are in the habit of provoking your significant other to a violent rage in the kitchen, you may have to worry about the enraged overhand icepick grip that some people say never happens.

That's the physical stuff. Gush exercise is really just a reminder. It tells the students that there is more to this, to anything we train, than just the motion.

Is gush emotional preparation for using a knife in self-defense? Not even close. It's a can of cherry cola wrapped in meat. It doesn't scream or writhe or convulse. It has no eyes. The smell is not and can never be right.

Is it icky? Yeah, and that's a start. A little nasty is always good for training. But it is a far, far cry from complete. It's a rush because the student is not expecting it. It can bring out a glitch if and when a student hesitates on the unexpected sensation—because when physical defense is triggered, especially if you are using a knife (which means lethal force is justified, which means lethal force is absolutely necessary right this second), you cannot afford to hesitate. Not even for a second.

Details:

- There are live knives involved. You need to have specific safety protocols for any drills with live knives. The protocols need to include minimum distances, safety officers, and a safe word that freezes all action.

- If you do this exercise, do it at the end of a day of hard training. That allows you to tell the students to wear clothes they don't mind getting destroyed without giving away that the instructions are for this exercise. The blood and cola stains probably aren't coming out.

- Don't use diet cola. It isn't sticky enough. Make sure it is warm, warmer than body temperature. And shake it really well.
- Rinse the steaks off before you barbecue them.

AFTERWORD

Real Superpowers You Can Have Today
(Send no money now, 90-day free trial on all Superpowers!
Change your life at no risk to you!)

- **Paying Attention to What You Are Doing:** This power makes you a force to be reckoned with, a model of efficiency. Something, especially on the highways and byways of our world, unique and effective.

- **Finishing the Hard Stuff First:** Normal humans stand staring with jaws open as you walk away from a job well done while they are still twiddling their thumbs, making coffee, and getting ready. You work out as they get ready to think about working out.

- **Really Listening:** For most people, a conversation is just a shallow attempt at getting their own ego stroked by people just as self-centered. With this superpower you can gather information, learn things, make friends, and be considered wise, intelligent, and caring.

- **Getting Off Your Ass and Doing Stuff:** We have superpowers to get stuff done, right? But even with superpowers, we actually have to get off our asses and do things. Act. This superpower not only allows you to get stuff done, the purpose of all superpowers, but by doing stuff you *learn things*. You *get experience*. This super-power, over time, gives you other superpowers! How is that fair?

- **Being Nice to People:** A subtle superpower that allows you to make friends, alleviate suffering, and even be proud of yourself.

- **Saying What You Mean:** One of the most dangerous superpowers, this two-edged sword can make any group you work with more efficient, but may make normals uncomfortable. Its complementary power, **Meaning What You Say**, has surprising force.

Superpowers within the reach of everyone. Try one today!

Really, people. Right there. Give it a try. They're free.

Please?

ACKNOWLEDGMENTS

It's been over thirty years of training, and I'm absolutely sure I'm going to miss somebody.

George Mattson, who wrote a description of ippon kumite that I completely misunderstood, resulting in the one-step drill.

Mike Moore and Wolfgang Dill, who set my martial base.

Dave Sumner, the best instructor I've had. I can never thank him enough. And his core of seniors, especially Harry Ford and Paul Bedard (sometimes the most dangerous man at the seminar is running the camera).

Paul McRedmond, the old silverback.

Lt. Howard Webb, who taught me the basics of doing scenarios. And the late Tim Bown and MG for pushing it a little further.

The MCSO Training Unit and CERT, for never accepting less than my best. And Sgt. (now Lieutenant) Jose Martinez, for seeing the need to rethink training, allowing us to create a program that dropped the injury rate by around 30 percent. Strange what happens when you let people who know what you need design what you use.

Maija Soderholm, the one who challenged me to write this all down. Deep thanks.

And, as always, Kami. The reason for everything.

BIBLIOGRAPHY

E. G. Bartlett: *Judo and Self-Defence* (New York: Thorsons Publishers, 1962).

Tony Blauer: tonyblauer.com.

Loren W. Christensen's works.

Michael Clarke: *The Art of Hojo Undo* (Wolfeboro: YMAA, 2009).

Jack Dempsey: *Championship Fighting: Explosive Punching and Aggressive Defense* (New York: Prentice-Hall, 1950).

Syd Hoare: *A–Z of Judo* (London: Ippon Books, 1994).

Keith Johnstone: *Impro: Improvisation and the Theatre* (New York: Routledge/Theatre Arts Books, 1981).

Rudyard Kipling: *Kim* (London: Macmillan, 1901).

Dave Lowry: *Autumn Lightning: The Education of an American Samurai* (Boston: Shambhala, 2001).

George E. Mattson: *The Way of Karate* (Rutland: Charles E. Tuttle, 1963).

National Child Traumatic Stress Network and National Center for PTSD: *Psychological First Aid: Field Operations Guide* (Los Angeles: NCTSN National Resource Center, 2006).

GLOSSARY

asocial. Interactions in which one or more of the people are not treating each other as people. Predators, for instance, will commonly treat victims as either resources or toys.

assault. A sudden attack with the intent of overwhelming the victim.

assumptions. Things that an instructor or practitioner believes. I believe most attacks happen at very close range. This assumption drives my bias as an infighter.

awareness. Knowledge of what is happening around you. Includes perception and understanding.

biases. Things an individual prefers. An instructor who prefers striking to grappling has a striking bias. I have an infighting bias.

bokken. "Wooden sword." A training katana.

center of gravity. The point at which one's entire body would balance—front to back, head to toes, and side to side.

coaching. Improving the performance of individuals.

dan tian. "Elixir field." The lower dan tian is the center of gravity.

deadly force. Legal term, exact definition varies by jurisdiction. Generally, force that can cause (or is intended to cause) death or "great bodily harm."

debriefing. A system for processing an event after the fact.

defense of a third party. Legal term for force used to defend someone other than yourself.

defensive tactics (DTs). Common law enforcement term for unarmed self-defense and restraint.

drop step. A technique for using uninhibited falling body weight as a power and speed enhancer.

facilitator. In scenario training, the instructor with primary responsibility for running the scenario and debriefing the student.

feeds. Fake attacks. Motion from a partner that mimics an attack but usually lacks the necessary elements to do any harm.

fighting. A give-and-take combative contest between two or more people.

ghosting. Using one's posture to induce the opponent to misread range.

gi. Traditional judo or karate uniform.

glitches. Internal hesitations, blind spots, and unconscious limitations.

hara. Belly. Center of gravity.

heart. Shorthand for the psychological, emotional, and spiritual elements that make one a good fighter or survivor.

initiative. The ability to move decisively and without hesitation.

intent. In threat assessment, intent is the will to cause you harm, to cause a third party harm, or to break any law that is your duty to enforce.

kumite. Karate sparring.

maai. Range. Distance and distance assessment.

means. In threat assessment, means is the physical ability to cause you harm, to cause a third party harm, or to break any law that is your duty to enforce.

mokuroku. "Certificate of full transmission" in some traditional Japanese systems.

MPDS. Movement, pain, damage, shock. The four classes of effects.

nage waza. Throwing techniques.

one-offs. Tricks or demonstrations that have a valuable lesson when first seen, but are not worth practicing regularly.

OODA loop. Col. John Boyd's model for decision-making. Observe, orient, decide, act.

operant conditioning. Training method for bringing a simple response to a stimulus to near-reflex speed.

opportunity. In threat assessment, opportunity is the ability to reach with the means to cause you harm, to cause a third party harm or to break any law that is your duty to enforce.

peer jury. A panel of fellow students who act as judges on the performance of the student.

permission. The ability to break one's social conditioning.

preclusion. In threat assessment, preclusion is the inability to do anything other than use physical force to prevent a threat from causing you harm, or causing a third party harm.

precursor movements. The motions a threat makes before he or she attacks (e.g., shifting weight, glancing away, or grabbing on to index a strike).

role player. An actor in scenario training.

safety briefing. Detailed instructions presented at the start of training to minimize injury and danger.

safety flaws. Artificial adaptations within drills and techniques to keep students from hurting themselves or each other.

safety officer. In scenario training, the instructor primarily responsible for safety. In all training, anyone and everyone responsible for safety is a safety officer. Everyone is a safety officer.

sambo. Russian martial art.

self-defense. Legal term for force used to protect one's self from immediate danger.

sensitivity drill. An exercise designed to increase the student's ability to gather and assess information.

social. Interactions in which the people treat each other as people.

social conditioning. Learned limits on our own behavior.

sparring. An exercise in fighting with very specific rules and usually designed to limit injury. Play fighting.

Spetsnaz. Russian special-operations units.

stop-action critique. Correcting a student by making the student freeze in place and then explaining what the instructor saw.

stress inoculation. Exposure to high-stress training in order to get one inured to the hormonal effects of high-stress environments.

sutemi waza. Sacrifice throws. Throwing techniques in which you throw yourself to the ground in order to force your opponent into a fall.

tanto. A Japanese-style combat knife.

teaching. Specifically, transmitting skill or knowledge through words or symbols.

threat. The bad guy.

threat assessment. An evaluation of the type and amount of danger a threat or situation represents.

threat profile. An assessment of the type of attacks one is likely to face.

tori. The one who demonstrates the technique in a partner drill. The defender.

training. Specifically, transmitting skill through repetitious action.

uke. One upon whom the technique is demonstrated. The attacker.

ukemi. The art of falling safely.

Violence Prone Play Group (VPPG). A group of senior practitioners who get together to explore and experiment.

woofing. Using aggressive and insulting talk to adrenalize and emotionally unbalance a student.

yoko ukemi. Side breakfall.

INDEX

ABOUT THE AUTHOR

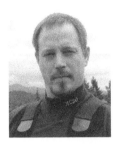

Rory Miller is a seventeen-year veteran of a metropolitan correctional system. He spent seventeen years, including ten as a sergeant, with the Multnomah County Sheriff's Office in Portland, Oregon. His assignments included booking, maximum security, disciplinary and administrative segregation, and mental health units. He was a CERT (Corrections Emergency Response Team) member for over eleven years and team leader for six.

His training has included over eight hundred hours of tactical training; witness protection and close-quarters handgun training with the local US Marshals; incident command system; instructor development courses; AELE discipline and internal investigations; hostage negotiations and hostage survival; integrated use of force and confrontational simulation instructor; mental health; defensive tactics, including the GRAPLE instructor program; diversity; and supervision.

Rory has designed and taught courses including confrontational simulations, uncontrolled environments, crisis communications with the mentally ill, CERT operations and planning, defensive tactics, and use of force.

In 2008 Rory Miller left his agency to spend over a year in Iraq with the Department of Justice ICITAP program as a civilian advisor to the Iraqi corrections system.

He has a bachelor's degree in psychology, a black belt in jujutsu, and college varsities in judo and fencing. He also likes long walks on the beach.

His writings have been featured in Loren Christensen's *Fighter's Fact Book 2: Street Fighting Essentials*, as well as Kane and Wilder's *Little Black Book of Violence* and *The Way to Black Belt*.

Rory is the author of *Meditations on Violence: A Comparison of Martial Arts Training & Real World Violence*, published by YMAA; *Violence: A Writer's Guide*, published by Smashwords; and *Facing Violence, Force Decisions*, and *Conflict Communication* published by YMAA.

BOOKS FROM YMAA

continued on next page . . .

DVDS FROM YMAA

more products available from . . .
YMAA Publication Center, Inc. 楊氏東方文化出版中心
1-800-669-8892 • info@ymaa.com • www.ymaa.com

CPSIA information can be obtained
at www.ICGtesting.com
Printed in the USA
LVHW032046281021
701855LV00002B/3